More Praise for *Cybermedicine*

"Informed and entertaining."
—*San Francisco Chronicle*

"Slack makes a well-reasoned case for the increased use of computers, both to help patients become more informed and, in some cases, to assist in their care."
—*Denver Post*

"An important book that will help all of us physicians to understand how computers can help us become more able, effective, and knowing doctors."
—Robert Coles, M.D., professor of psychiatry and medical humanities, Harvard Medical School and winner of the Pulitzer Prize

"This highly readable book should attract anyone interested in the computer medical revolution."
—Alvan R. Feinstein, M.D., Sterling Professor of Medicine & Epidemiology, Yale University School of Medicine

"This is not a book about bits and bytes, but an appraisal of the computer's current role in health care and how its future will be defined."
—Peter Goldman, M.D., Maxwell Finland Professor of Clinical Pharmacology Emeritus, Harvard Medical School

Cybermedicine

Warner V. Slack, M.D.

Cartoons by Charles Slack

Cybermedicine

How Computing Empowers
Doctors and Patients for Better Care
Revised and Updated Edition

With a Foreword by Ralph Nader

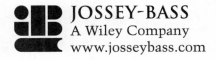

JOSSEY-BASS
A Wiley Company
www.josseybass.com

Published by

JOSSEY-BASS
A Wiley Company
350 Sansome St.
San Francisco, CA 94104-1342

www.josseybass.com

Jossey-Bass books and products are available through most bookstores. To contact Jossey-Bass directly, call (888) 378-2537, fax to (800) 605-2665, or visit our website at www.josseybass.com.

Substantial discounts on bulk quantities of Jossey-Bass books are available to corporations, professional associations, and other organizations. For details and discount information, contact the special sales department at Jossey-Bass.

We at Jossey-Bass strive to use the most environmentally sensitive paper stocks available to us. Our publications are printed on acid-free recycled stock whenever possible, and our paper always meets or exceeds minimum GPO and EPA requirements.

Library of Congress Cataloging-in-Publication Data

Slack, Warner V., date
  Cybermedicine : how computing empowers doctors and patients for better care / Warner V. Slack ; with a foreword by Ralph Nader.—Rev. and updated ed.
      p. ; cm.
Includes bibliographical references and index.
  ISBN 0-7879-5631-7 (alk. paper)
1. Medical informatics. 2. Physician and patient. [DNLM: 1. Medical Informatics Applications. 2. Physician-Patient Relations. 3. Practice Management, Medical.
W26.5 S631c 2001] I. Title.
  R858 .S556 2001
  610'.285—dc21   2001002782

SECOND EDITION
PB Printing 10 9 8 7 6 5 4 3 2 1

—ᴗᴗ— Contents

For Carolyn

—⚋— Foreword

Cybermedicine is a book resting on a seeming paradox—a very compassionate, patient-first physician pressing for bolder and more comprehensive computer uses in clinical medicine and in direct patient interaction. Dr. Warner V. Slack, a pioneer in clinical computing (starting in the 1960s at the University of Wisconsin Medical School and later at the Center for Clinical Computing and Harvard Medical School), argues in this work that there is no necessary paradox at all, if the evolution of computers in medicine adheres to what is best for patients and their enhanced role as decision makers.

And what are the guidelines that would enable the computer to have "a humanizing influence on the practice of medicine" and "help patients and their families maintain better health, manage medical problems when they occur, seek and use health care facilities in an enlightened manner, and participate as partners with clinicians in medical decisions that can both improve the quality and reduce the cost of medical care"? There are nine, according to Dr. Slack. Before the programs become widespread, "They should be medically sound; they should be easy to use; they should be truly interactive; they should be of immediate and if possible long-range benefit to the patient; they should have the patient in charge; they should protect confidentiality; they should be readily available to people of all socioeconomic backgrounds; they should be fast and reliable; and they should be studied for effectiveness and safety." However comprehensive, these standards do represent a tall order, especially given the stigmas, phobias, and computer illiteracy that impede a clear highway in the minds of many. Especially given those hospital bureaucracies and administrative myopias, which Dr. Slack, putting on his estimable literary scrubs, dissects and parodies mercilessly near the end of the book in a brilliant finale, graced by a poignant description of his young diabetic grandson.

What is so attractive about *Cybermedicine* is that Dr. Slack is no gee-whiz technophile, breathlessly promoting a scenario of inevitable technology for a brave new world of diagnosis, treatment, prevention, and self-help. He permeates his book with continual skepticism in order to discipline his enthusiasm. And well he might, knowing, as he demonstrates, the past failures, overpromises, misuses, and dehumanizations of other technologies, including more than a few of the medical variety. But he also knows that inventors and early developers of communications and computer technologies often underpredicted both their uses and their impact—sometimes stunningly so in retrospect.

Over twenty years ago, I convened the first conference on computers and the consumer. Even at that time, it was apparent that computers were receiving a highly one-sided application on the side of manufacturers, wholesalers, and retail vendors. The consumer was neither getting direct access to this new tool nor receiving direct benefits such as easily retrievable data on comparative prices, safety, durability, and other product and service data in order to shop more wisely. Indeed, sellers were accumulating more and more data about consumers—medical, credit, buying patterns, and so on—which also invaded their privacy.

The still one-sided applications of computers pertain to medicine as well. The inventory, administrative, billing, and patient records sections of hospitals, for example, have computers with more and more complex software to serve the vendors, euphemistically called the providers. Dr. Slack wants the computer programs in these more mundane areas, along with the direct interface between clinicians and patients, to be placed for use by and at the service of patients and their families. A particularly prominent illustration of one-sided computerization is computerized billing fraud and abuse, which one General Accounting Office report estimated to be consuming 10 percent of health care expenditures in this country. Imagine the discipline that would result from more consumer-side use of and access to computerized data and practices in billing, medical malpractice, budgetary allocations between clinical and administrative personnel, and other festering conditions in America's largest industry, which will reach one trillion dollars in 1997.

The human factors approach to technology, as with automotive safety, has registered major declines in mortality and morbidity in recent decades. Dr. Slack believes that enough has now been demon-

strated, as described in this book, to warrant an accelerated and comprehensive advance in clinical computing in hospitals and clinics, leading to direct patient and family use of interactive computer programs
that have human beings at the other end to ensure the supremacy of
the patient's needs. As he writes, "Any doctor who can be replaced by
a computer deserves to be." Because computerized business and professional cultures can become interminably fascinating ends in themselves, it is obligatory for practitioners of clinical computing to ask,
and measure the results from answering, these questions: "Is the computer helping to improve the quality of medical care? Is the computer
helping the patient in matters of health and illness?"

Cybermedicine does not duck the "but" issues; it faces them forth-
rightly, as in the discussion of privacy and confidentiality. It stresses
trying, testing, and revising as built-in cautions against wrongheaded
turns or computer hubris.

The growing domination of conglomerate-directed managed care,
with its control of practitioners, its de-skilling of staff, and its shifting
of costs onto the consumer, presents new imperatives for patient
empowerment. Enter more home care. In a recent report on the new
asthma care guidelines issued by the National Heart, Lung, and Blood
Institute of the National Institutes of Health, asthma patients were
urged to take more control of their own treatment. "Medicine is a
partnership now," said Dr. Shirley Murphy, a professor at the University of New Mexico school of medicine and chairperson of the experts
panel. "Patients need to take a greater responsibility for managing
their chronic disease." There will be more such urgings for patient self-
management.

Notwithstanding its thematic optimism and concrete justifications,
Cybermedicine does not underestimate the obstacles nor the unin-
tended consequences of interactions between and among computers,
clinicians, and patients. There is a long road ahead, in the midst of
episodic progress, before this machine and its software are made to
adjust to human beings at all levels and backgrounds. This book ele-
vates the discussion and the search for greater heights of public
scrutiny and evaluation, and does so in a clear, at times literary, style.
And it is style that puts substance on wheels.

Washington, D.C.   RALPH NADER
March 1997

—ᗡᗡ— New Preface

Shortly after the Second World War, the eminent mathematician Norbert Wiener drew upon the Greek word *kybernetes,* meaning "pilot" or "governor," to coin the English word *cybernetics,* which he defined as the science of communication between people and machines. More recently, the word *cyberspace* has come to mean the worldwide computer-based network that already has so greatly enhanced communication. And as a derivative of cybernetics, *cybermedicine* is our word for what in the past my colleagues and I have called "clinical computing": the use of computing to enhance communication in the field of medicine. For the most part, I will use *cybermedicine* in lieu of "clinical computing" (or what is often called "medical informatics") in the text of this new edition.

Only three years have passed since the first publication of *Cybermedicine* in 1997, but these years have seen a remarkable proliferation of medical information on the Internet. By a recent poll, approximately sixty million people in the United States signed on to the Internet to look up medically related information. As for American physicians, another poll indicated that on average close to 90 percent of them go on-line to the Internet, and over 50 percent are daily users. In the pages that follow, I have expanded the chapters titled "The Patient On-Line" and "The Clinician On-Line" to include a discussion of this greatly expanded use. There are a number of recent reference guides to health-related information on the Internet for both clinician and patient, and I have listed a representative sample of these in the bibliography for this preface.

In spite of the rapid acceleration of on-line usage, however, good cybermedicine is still more the exception than the rule, and the chapter now called "Barriers to Cybermedicine" is as apt today as it was when I first wrote it. But since the consultant as a barrier to good cybermedicine deserves special attention, I have given this topic its own chapter, "The Importance of Being Ernst." I have also added to the discussions of how to evaluate cybermedicine and my hopes for the future, and given them new chapters titled "How Well Does It Work?" and "New Horizons." Finally, I have gone through the entire book in the effort to update and improve the content of *Cybermedicine* in ways consistent with these changing times.

Most writers have a little narcissism in them. Putting words on paper (or in a machine) implies the hope if not the expectation that someone will read them—not necessarily like them but at least read them. Much of what is in this little book has been published previously. Whether this will be read anew, or reread, or in either case found worthwhile, I can only hope.

For those of you who would like to read on, a word of caution. I come to this book not as a disinterested observer but as one immersed in the field, with a personal perspective and with opinions not necessarily shared by others. Some are controversial, and some *quite* controversial—even to the point of evoking an occasional expression of alarm from a publisher here and there (a lot of support as well, it should be mentioned) and an occasional expression of anger from a reader.

As with all good publishers, Jossey-Bass made it clear to me at the start that I would have the final say about what appears in *Cybermedicine,* and I must assume responsibility for the content. I might add, however, that this proviso implies a bit of arrogance, as if the ideas not specifically attributed to others are necessarily original with me. I know only too well the possibility that others have contributed ideas that, with fallible and, although I hope not, *selective* memory, I have incorporated into my intellectual lexicon and presented as my own. So to any whose unacknowledged ideas have become part of this book, I extend both my apologies and thanks.

ACKNOWLEDGMENTS

I am deeply indebted to my parents, Evelyn and Charles, my children—Alison, Charles (the real writer in the family, who also did the cartoons for the book), and Jennifer—and their families, and most of all my wife, Carolyn, for all their help and support.

I want to give special thanks to Emily Boro, editor in residence in the Center for Clinical Computing. Emily has been of invaluable help to me with my writing over the years. She has edited many of the articles that I have incorporated into my book, and she has helped me in immeasurable ways with the entire manuscript. I also want to thank Alan Rinzler, my excellent editor at Jossey-Bass, and Lisa Underhill for her editorial assistance with this edition of *Cybermedicine.* And I want to thank Robert McCarty and his colleagues at RJM Associates and Donna Safran in the Center for Clinical Computing for their superb documentary video of our cybermedicine systems.

I am greatly indebted to John Cameron of the University of Wisconsin, who welcomed me into his laboratory and gave me support and wise counsel when I first decided to pursue cybermedicine, and to Frank Larson and Robert Schilling of the University of Wisconsin, Morris Collen of the Kaiser Permanente Hospitals, Raymond Keating of the Mayo Clinic, and Alvan R. Feinstein of Yale University School of Medicine for their support and guidance in my early years of cybermedicine. I am also indebted to the past chairmen of my departments, A. Stone Freedberg, Howard Frazier, and Franklin Epstein of the Department of Medicine at Beth Israel Hospital, Eugene Braunwald of the Consolidated Department of Medicine at Beth Israel and Brigham and Women's hospitals, and Freddy Frankel, of the Department of Psychiatry at Beth Israel Hospital, for their support and encouragement over the years. And I am indebted to Mitchell T. Rabkin and David Dolins of Beth Israel Hospital, and Richard Nesson and Anthony Komaroff of Brigham and Women's Hospital, for inviting us into their hospitals and giving us the mandate and means to develop our cybermedicine systems.

I want also to give special thanks to my colleagues Phillip Hicks, Hollis Kowaloff, Douglas Porter, and Lawrence Van Cura who have contributed in immeasurable ways to my research with patient-computer dialogue, and to Robert Beckley, who has provided outstanding technical leadership in cybermedicine over the years at both Beth Israel Deaconess Medical Center and Brigham and Women's Hospital.

I am particularly grateful to Howard Hiatt, an early staunch supporter of cybermedicine at Harvard Medical School and my esteemed mentor over the years; to my brother, Charles, my best friend and valued colleague; and to Howard Bleich, my partner in our center for over thirty years and a true pioneer in cybermedicine.

And finally, I am indebted to my friends and colleagues at the Center for Clinical Computing, Beth Israel Deaconess Medical Center, Brigham and Women's Hospital, Harvard Medical School, and the University of Wisconsin, for their many contributions to the work described in this book.

Boston, Mass.   WARNER V. SLACK, M.D.
June 2001

⟶ Preface to First Edition

When I was in medical school in the late 1950s, I was troubled by the emphasis on memorization. It was as if we novice doctors were expected to keep all the information necessary to practice good medicine in our minds at all times, never forgetting anything for a moment. Notes and reminders were frowned on. I also remember that the *Merck Manual* fit nicely in the pocket of my white jacket and that old Professor Gradgrind accosted me with critical countenance and words of derision for carrying it, as if looking something up were a form of cheating. Yet the professor's professed expectations seemed inconsistent with the workings of the human brain—rapid, reliable recall of a large number of facts is not its forte—so, along with my classmates, I quickly learned to do my looking up in private. (A curious ritual in college had led many of us to pretend we hadn't studied for a test when we really had, in order to appear "intelligent" to our peers.)

It also seemed clear to me that this obsession with memory was not good for patients, particularly since we were destined to work with a rapidly expanding base of information. What if I forgot something? I thought of the airline pilot who was thoroughly familiar with the instruments in the cockpit yet still had to go through a checklist (an aeronautical *Merck Manual,* so to speak) before takeoff and landing. And as a passenger, I was reassured by the process. I decided that I would want my doctor to look things up. It was then that I first had the idea that the computer, which was just coming into being, could be of help to doctors and patients in the future of medicine.

Later, as a resident in neurology and then on the faculty, I had the good fortune to spend the decade of the 1960s at the University of Wisconsin in Madison, where a wonderfully radical atmosphere of strong social conscience and progressive ideology pervaded the campus. Remarkable science was being done there as well. John Cameron was doing pioneering work in medical physics, Gobind Khorana was synthesizing a gene in a test tube, Robert Schilling was breaking new ground in hematology, Frank Larson and Phillip Hicks were revolutionizing laboratory medicine, Charles Heidelberger was pioneering new approaches to chemotherapy for cancer, Howard Temin was postulating reverse transcriptase in RNA viruses, Milton Yatvin was lending new understanding to the hormonal control of genetic expression, Harry Harlow was elucidating the psychological bonds between mother and infant, and Carl Rogers, in a small, two-story cottage on University Avenue, was developing his theory of non-directive psychotherapy.

It was in this environment that two lines of reasoning evolved in my mind. The first was that the computer could be used wisely and well in the practice of medicine. The electronic digital computer, with its capacity to hold large amounts of data and to execute multiple complex instructions with great speed and accuracy, would, I reasoned, find an important clinical role in both diagnosis and treatment. Why couldn't the computer satisfy the need for facts and free the doctor to spend more time with the existentially important aspects of the doctor-patient relationship? The idea was controversial, and those of us who were entering this new field were confronted by concerns about the computer in medicine under any circumstances. Would these machines result in the dehumanizing processes that had been associated with the industrial revolution? Would modern times destroy the art of medicine?

The second line of reasoning led to a philosophy that I called "patient power," in the vernacular of the times, arguing that patients who want to should be encouraged to make their own clinical decisions and helped to do so. For centuries, the medical profession had perpetrated paternalism as an essential component of medical care, thereby depriving patients of the self-esteem that comes from self-reliance and mutual respect. The assumption was that the doctor knew best. Patient power questioned this assumption. As George Bernard Shaw once wrote, "Do not do unto others as you would that they should do unto you. Their tastes may not be the same."

Like the idea of computers in medicine, the idea of patient power was highly controversial for its time. In 1961, during a visit to our home in Madison, my brother, Charles, took me to meet Carl Rogers, who had introduced the concept of client-centered therapy to clinical psychology. This meeting was one of the turning points in my life.

Rogers's support of patient power was the reinforcement I needed to persevere.

Contrary to the prevailing wisdom of the 1960s, the computer was destined to play an important role in patient power. In dialogue with the patient, the computer would be a means of transferring control to the patient, a "patient's assistant" if you will. And in dialogue with the doctor and other clinicians who care for patients, the computer would be a helpful extension of the mind. Contrary to the dire predictions of well-meaning humanists, the computer would have a *humanizing* influence on the practice of medicine.

There were to be two developments that would augment the interaction between patient and computer and between clinician and computer. One was the Internet. I did not know it at the time, but in the 1960s, the seeds of the Internet, which would revolutionize worldwide communication, were beginning to germinate. The other development was the personal computer. During the same thirty-year period beginning in the 1960s, the computer was to evolve from a large, expensive, cumbersome mainframe to a small, affordable, easy-to-use personal machine.

Today, patients with PCs and access to the Internet no longer have to depend on the medical establishment for information on health and disease. They can sign on at any time of day or night, read medical articles, and communicate with other patients. Clinicians are also availing themselves of the medical information available on the Internet and the ability to communicate by e-mail. Furthermore, clinicians and patients are using e-mail to communicate with each other, exchanging information and offering advice and suggestions as peers, in a manner unprecedented in the annals of medicine. This is patient power at work, fostered by computer technology.

———

My argument in this book is that computer programs that help patients and doctors with medical matters can both improve the quality and reduce the cost of medical care. Programs that help the doctor practice medicine can also improve the quality of the doctor's working life. In addition, good cybermedicine can improve the relationship between the patient and doctor.

Yet good cybermedicine is still more the exception than the rule, particularly in those hospitals and clinics where bureaucracy prevails.

Ironically, with the burgeoning technology of worldwide communications, doctors and patients often have more computing available to them outside the walls of their medical institutions than inside them.

In spite of the great advances in computer technology, the clinician, the patient, and the prospective patient have yet to realize the full benefit of these machines. There are of course real dangers with the misuse of the computer, such as true dehumanization, depersonalization, and breach of privacy, and we must keep our guard up. On balance, however, the problem is not too much computing in medicine; the problem is *too little*.

—*w*—

In the pages that follow, I discuss my experience with computers in medicine over the past thirty-five years. And on the basis of this experience, I offer suggestions for the future. This is not a review of the uses of the computer in medicine. (I would suggest Morris Collen's *A History of Medical Informatics in the United States, 1950 to 1990* as an excellent review of the field.) I refer only briefly to the work of others, although I am well aware that my voice is but one among many. This is one individual's account, based on personal experience. If my experiences with cybermedicine produce even a little optimism in your mind about the future of medicine, an important goal will have been accomplished. And if you come to realize what the forces of bureaucracy are doing to reduce the quality of that future—and what clinicians and concerned patients can have if they insist on computing that puts their interests ahead of administrative careerism—then my book will have served its purpose.

Boston, Mass.   WARNER V. SLACK, M.D.
January 1997

Cybermedicine

PART ONE

Cybermedicine and the Patient

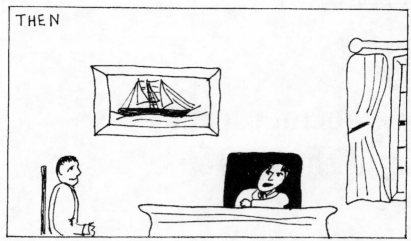

THEN

"I THINK THERE IS A WORLD MARKET FOR MAYBE FIVE COMPUTERS."
THOMAS WATSON, CHAIRMAN, IBM, 1943

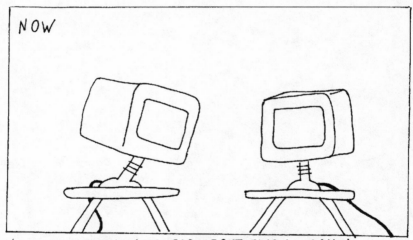

NOW

"I FORESEE THE NEED FOR ABOUT FIVE HUMANS."

CHAPTER ONE

Providing Information to Patients

I t can be argued that the largest yet most neglected health care resource, worldwide, is the patient or prospective patient. Most people could readily manage a number of common, important medical problems, such as sore throat and urinary tract infection, if provided with the clinical information necessary to do so. I don't mean to suggest that self-care can be accomplished by taking Hygiene 101 from the basketball coach in his spare time—or by studying Molecular Biology 401, with a discourse on the genetic determinants of immunological mechanisms. I mean good, solid, reliable, up-to-date, best current wisdom that virtually any literate person who wants to can understand.

Until recently, communication between doctor and patient was for the most part one-way—the doctor ordered and the patient was expected to obey. The "good" patient followed orders dutifully; the noncompliant (read "bad") patient didn't. But times are changing; not as fast as we might like, but changing for the better.

It has long been my argument that doctors should give people sufficient information to enable them, or their designated surrogates, to make enlightened decisions about matters of health and disease. People should know how they can best achieve and preserve good health and the good health of their families. They should know when a problem is not a medical problem—when, for example, the sadness that follows the loss of a loved one is healthy grief that will abate with time, and when it is clinical depression that could benefit from counseling or medication. They should know when to care for a medical problem themselves and how best to do this—for example, how to care for a laceration that is too small for stitches (lots of soap and water, no iodine).

People also need to know when it would be better to turn to others for help and how and where to do so. What are often the most difficult of diagnostic decisions typically get left to the patient—when to consult a doctor, which doctor to consult, and how to get in touch. When, for example, is the laceration big enough for stitches, and where should the stitching be done? In a medical emergency, people need to know what to do.

HOW DOCTORS TALK TO PATIENTS

Doctors can help people become better informed about matters of health and disease in a number of ways. The oldest and in many ways still the most effective medium is face-to-face communication. Dialogue between doctor and patient is the mainstay of clinical medicine. During the interpersonal encounter, the doctor tries to establish rapport, develop bonds of mutual respect and trust, collect information relevant to a patient's medical problems and general health, and communicate information for the patient's immediate and long-range use. In turn, the patient can explain his or her wishes to the doctor, and the two can work together to develop an approach to treatment consistent with both the patient's wishes and the dictates of medical science. Of course individual attention is not always possible, and when it is, it can be very expensive. Even in the best of circumstances, practicing physicians are faced with serious problems when it comes to dialogue with their patients. Clinical interviewing requires a large amount of time, and inadequate histories and insufficient counseling often result from limitations in time beyond the physician's control.

Since the Second World War, advances in medical care have outstripped our ability to apply them, and pressures on health care systems worldwide have escalated. Doctors are pressured on one hand by increasingly empowered patients, who understandably want and expect more personal attention, and on the other hand by parsimonious bureaucrats, who schedule more and more patients in shorter and shorter intervals. There is a pressing need, therefore, to seek new ways to enhance medical communication and thereby supplement the interpersonal relationship between doctor and patient. The idea is not to replace the doctor; the idea is to fill a void.

How then, can medical information be communicated in the absence of direct interpersonal communication?

Early Technology

Since early times, growth in population has been accompanied by innovation in communication, inventions that enhance the exchange of information between more and more people, but that do so at the expense of direct interpersonal conversation. Each invention, impersonal by its very nature, has in turn been subject to early criticism both by the well-meaning humanist, who objects to anything seen as having a depersonalizing influence, and by the well-meaning traditionalist, who opposes innovation on principle. It is likely that when that ingenious Sumerian who invented writing first pressed those cuneiform symbols into clay along the Tigris River some five thousand years ago, a skeptic standing nearby predicted with furrowed brow that people would soon stop *talking* to each other. Those who read *The Republic* in school will remember that Plato was very much opposed to theater as it was performed in ancient Greece. For him the portrayal of fictional characters was an ignoble pursuit that exposed audiences to the risk of corruption.

In more modern times, the telephone was written off prematurely: according to an internal memorandum at Western Union in 1876, the telephone "has too many shortcomings to be seriously considered as a means of communication. The device is inherently of no value to us." The motion picture was also greeted with suspicion. The stage was by then a reputable medium ("legitimate theater," as it were), but the movie, even as it gained in popularity, was deemed *common* and potentially harmful. To make a movie based on a book was a priori to debase the book. Parents worried about bad cinematic influences and meted out movie-going privileges with extreme judiciousness. Dorothy Parker likened the movie to sex, pointing out that while most enjoyed it, few would talk about it.

Radio had a similar history. "The wireless music box has no imaginable commercial value. Who would pay for a message sent to nobody in particular?" argued David Sarnoff's associates in the 1920s, when he urged them to support radio as a commercial venture. Popular as it was to become, radio was late to be accepted publicly by the intelligentsia. *The Green Hornet, Captain Midnight, Terry and the Pirates,* and *Superman* (together with their comic book counterparts) were intermittently banned from middle-class households. Kids, of course, still listened—but did so with youthful subterfuge.

After World War II came television—lowbrow (boxing and wrestling were the staple programs) and frowned upon as potentially corrupting. As television broadened its scope and became increasingly available and popular, it was correspondingly chic among the culturati *not* to have television at home. There was a family in our neighborhood in the 1970s who did not have a set in their home. Mention of television in conversation with the parents elicited blank faces. The children, however, spent an inordinate amount of time in front of *our* set.

Movies and radio were by then regarded as legitimate art forms, particularly the earlier, pre–World War II films and programs. It was then acceptable to consider a movie *better* than the book on which it was based (*Elmer Gantry* and *The Godfather* come to mind).

The personal computer is the new medium on the block. And once again, prophecy was off the mark. "I think there is a world market for maybe five computers," Thomas Watson, chairman of IBM, is purported to have said in 1943. But I am getting ahead of myself.

Medicine and the Printed Word

When Johannes Gutenberg invented the printing press in the mid-fifteenth century, he used his invention to publish the first printed version of the Christian Bible. His machine of course would have an enormous influence on secular communication, but the medical profession would be slow to adopt the printed word as a means of communication with patients. Patients were to be kept in the dark, knowing only what their doctors wanted them to know. Information in the hands of the patient could be dangerous, it was believed. When the doctor handed the patient a prescription it was written in Latin to *prevent* communication. Well into the twentieth century, medical articles in the popular press were treated at best with amusement by the profession. This reluctance to go public with professional secrets is not unique to medicine. Most professions are protective of their information, which serves to differentiate them from the public. Scientists who write for the public risk criticism from their peers; only giants such as Einstein can write for the nonscientist without at least some risk of reprisal from the scientific priesthood. To this day, doctors who write for the public are vulnerable to the criticism of publicity seeking, of pandering to the public and jeopardizing the patient, for whom it is argued a little knowledge might be a dangerous thing. The concern that the public will not understand and will be misled is certainly legitimate, but it is sometimes expressed as a covert means of protecting the guild, rather than the public. There is valuable equity in the concentration of information within a profession.

In 1946 came a turning point in medical publications for the public. Pocket Books published *Baby and Child Care*, by Benjamin Spock. Criticized at first by the American Medical Association and the American Psychological Association—for pandering to the public, being too permissive in approach, and definitely *not* representing Park Avenue pediatrics—Spock's book so obviously filled a niche that it could not be stifled. It told how to care for a sick baby at 2 A.M.; it told parents when they could care for the baby at home and when to call a doctor, when to worry and when *not* to worry. Parents might not discuss Spock's advice at a seminar on psychological theory or at a golf club social, but there was no way that *anyone* was going to wrest Spock's book from their hands when their child was sick. It has been estimated that *Baby and Child Care* is second only to the Bible in total sales. Spock went a long way toward legitimizing the medical book for the public, and publications on self-care are now published in abundance, many even with the blessing of the AMA. The adage that "the person who treats himself has a fool for a doctor" is being replaced by titles such as *How to Be Your Own Doctor*.

Yet the published forum, like the lecture, is still a type of one-way communication. There is little provision for interaction with the author or lecturer. In addition, it can be hard to assess the accuracy of published material—particularly if experts disagree, which is often the case in the medical profession (more often than we care to acknowledge). When there is disagreement, whose advice does the reader follow? One cannot turn readily to the writer and ask for evidence. Still, a book can be kept close at hand, available for quick reference whenever needed, at any time of day or night.

As self-help books and articles on medical matters appear at an accelerating rate, their success creates a bewildering surfeit. The problem now is how to select the ones that can be trusted. And most of us cannot afford to house large libraries in our homes. Even when a good book is at hand, locating the desired chapter or page may be hard, even with an index and table of contents.

The ideal would be to have Dr. Spock in conversation in the living room. But to have his words of wisdom on the printed page, close at hand, is still a good alternative, impersonal as it may be. Books are portable and are usually replaceable if lost or worn out. The first-aid manual is here to stay, at least for the foreseeable future. Still, the health-minded reader can be left hanging with important questions.

The Airwaves

Perhaps recognizing the problems of books, a few doctors have turned to the airwaves, sometimes reluctantly and sometimes with zeal. As far back as 1936, CBS radio aired a fifteen-minute child health program, hosted by Dr. Alan Roy Dafoe, the physician who delivered the Dionne quintuplets. But radio and television are still basically one-way communicators over which the listener has little control. With medical topics, it is the producer and not the patient who schedules the programming. A diabetic in need of immediate advice is not going to tune in to a lengthy discussion of intermediary glucose metabolism on public television if a booklet from the American Diabetes Association is readily available on the kitchen shelf.

In some radio and television programs, however, the listener or viewer can converse with the expert over the telephone. This type of talk show is a response, I'm convinced, to the frustration evoked by one-way communication. People are restless by nature; they like to interact. They can take just so much of Pat Robertson without wanting to talk back. (If you're itching to talk back to *me* at this moment, you can use my e-mail address: wslack@caregroup.harvard.edu.) And sit-still behavior does not come naturally. The ever-proliferating cellular phone (ubiquitous on streets from Sydney to Paris to New York) is another example of the guy on the street talking back.

The audience participation talk show was invented, almost certainly, not by a clever producer but by an irate listener who demanded the opportunity to get a word in, albeit edgewise. Sports and politics, the first call-in topics, still dominate the airwaves, but medicine has found its dial-in niche, whereby doctors can give specific advice to callers. On midday television in Boston, Timothy Johnson takes "house calls" on medical matters, Tom Cottle counsels troubled callers on psychological issues, and Alexis Beck gives advice on nutrition. In San Francisco, Dean Edell offers medical common sense on both radio and television call-in shows. Helpful as these programs may be, however, they still serve mainly as forums of general interest, rather than solutions to the specific medical needs of patients. The waiting time for callers is long, often as long as the time in the physician's waiting room, few callers get on the air, and airtime is short.

WHEN PATIENTS TALK WITH PATIENTS

In 1935, Bill W., a recovering alcoholic, found himself in Akron, Ohio, the victim of a failed business venture. Fearful that he might have a relapse, Bill had a remarkable insight—if he wanted to help himself, he should find and help another alcoholic. He found Dr. Bob, an alcoholic physician, and helped him to stop drinking. It was there, in Akron, that Bill W. and Dr. Bob (neither of whom ever drank again) founded Alcoholics Anonymous, the most successful approach to alcoholism ever devised.

Bill W.'s insight, that one's own experience with a medical problem can be used to help someone else with the same problem, and that in doing this, one is also helping oneself, is at the heart of all successful self-help and medical support programs. Only an alcoholic can fully understand the experience of alcoholism. Only a woman who has undergone a mastectomy for breast cancer herself can fully understand what is in store for another woman with the same diagnosis. Only the parents of a toddler with diabetes will know what this entails—the blood tests, insulin injections, meal planning, and day-to-day living, at home and in the outside world. And in communicating their experiences to help others, these people are putting their problems to good use in what I think is the most durable form of altruism—helping yourself by helping others. Sadly, the self-help programs in their early days were sometimes treated with scorn by the medical profession. But doctors are coming to realize, however belatedly, that all of us—patient and clinician alike—can benefit from the principle that patients and their families are an invaluable resource for one another. This is enlightened self-interest in the best sense of the term.

Initiated not by clinical experts but by people who share the same problem, symbiotic communication has seen remarkable growth over the past sixty-five years. More and more, people are sharing their problems and their strategies for coping, both formally and informally, one on one, in groups, forums, books, and pamphlets, and on radio and television. The wise doctor knows when *not* to intrude on such beneficial communication.

ON-THE-SPOT INSTRUCTION

It is helpful to differentiate between information that we need to commit to memory and information that is readily available through external sources. In the classroom, where great emphasis is placed on memory, external sources of information are suspect. Teachers worry about the handheld calculator or the use of crib notes during an examination. Outside the classroom, however, memory is less important. If information is on hand whenever needed—for example, how to start the furnace, how to place the jumper cables, or, on a more esoteric level, how to calculate the area under a curve—there is little need to memorize. There are even good reasons not to rely on memory.

Rapid, reliable recall is not always a strength of the human mind, for all its marvelous attributes. It is often safer to read instructions than to rely on memory, particularly when the information is important but rarely used. Paradoxically, if the information is often used, this too can result in errors. When the familiarity of a protocol leads to boredom, the mind tends to wander. When the stakes are high, as in the cockpit of a commercial airplane about to take off, the copilot reads a checklist to the pilot, even though the pilot knows the panel by heart.

And so it is in medicine, at least for the patient if not the doctor. Doctors tend to be obsessed with memory (knowing it all can be a matter of pride), although less so than in days gone by. But patients do not need to memorize medical information. They just need to have it handy. Better to have the first-aid manual readily available than to commit its contents to memory.

ENTER THE COMPUTER

The essence of the computer, in contrast to the book, play, movie, radio, or television, is its ability to *interact*, to converse with its user one on one. As a prescription for the patient, the computer can be programmed to simulate one-on-one conversation, but with the collective wisdom of many doctors.

The idea of a patient "talking" to a computer was hotly debated at its inception in the radical decade of the 1960s and is still controversial. This is understandable. Novelty is unsettling. It is hard for us to assess the potential, for good or for bad, of a new idea. This is true in virtually all walks of life—the arts, the sciences, the professions, and the marketplace. Good ideas are often thwarted. As Machiavelli observed, "The innovator makes enemies of all those who prospered under the old order." (Not all those with enemies are innovators, of course.)

And so it has been in medicine. On one hand, bad ideas are often promulgated. Carcinogenic X rays were once used to treat normal thymus glands, ringworm, and acne; tonsillectomies were routinely performed under general anesthesia in healthy children; and the operation to remove the frontal lobes of the brain (prefrontal lobotomy) was a common treatment for mental illness. On the other hand, René Laënnec was ridiculed for his invention of the stethoscope (it separated the doctor's ear from the patient's chest), and Ignaz Semmelweis couldn't convince his fellow Viennese obstetricians to wash their hands before delivery.

And so it has been with the invention of the computer and its introduction to society and medicine.

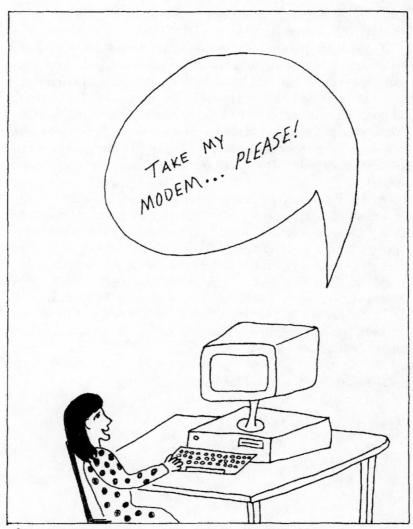

BREAKING THE ICE WITH A LITTLE HUMOR

CHAPTER TWO

Patient-Computer Dialogue

The first patient to "talk" to a computer did so at the University of Wisconsin Hospitals in 1965. At the time, my goal with the computer in medicine was to help the doctor with diagnosis and treatment. It was clear from the start, however, that if the computer was to help with the care of a patient, good information about the patient would have to be available to the computer—for example, the medical history, obtained from an interview with the patient, the physical examination, obtained by the doctor, and the results of diagnostic studies, obtained from the laboratory. My office mate, Philip Hicks, was working to automate the laboratories; I decided to start with the medical history.

The traditional method of taking and recording medical histories involves serious problems for the busy clinician, particularly in areas of our country that are short on doctors. Asking a lot of questions takes a lot of time, and incomplete histories frequently result from time limitations beyond the doctor's control. In the 1960s, northern Wisconsin was short of doctors; for those who were seeing up to thirty or forty patients a day, there was barely enough time to ask "Where does it hurt?"—let alone all the other questions in the standard interview.

Furthermore, recording the results of a medical interview in longhand was a laborious process, and histories were often nonstandardized, incomplete, and illegibly written—characteristics that greatly hampered the subsequent use of this information in patient care and clinical research.

At the time, self-administered paper questionnaires were being used with considerable success; the Cornell Medical Index and the "multiphasic" questionnaire of the Permanente Medical Group provided standardized, consistent, and inexpensive methods for taking medical histories. Furthermore, the Cornell and Permanente systems used a computer to process the responses—one of the first applications of the computer in medicine. And many good self-administered medical questionnaires are used throughout the country today. Questionnaires, however, cannot be tailored to the particular needs of the individual because they permit no interaction. They provide no mechanism either to clarify the meaning of a question or to qualify the answer. If the respondent answers the question, "Have you had any pain in your chest?" with "yes," it could mean a minor ache or impending heart trouble. The respondent might misunderstand a question (and thereby give an erroneous answer), inadvertently skip a question, or lose one or more pages of the questionnaire. Furthermore, filling out questionnaires is drudgery.

In my first attempt to overcome these problems, I borrowed from a method first developed by Morris Collen and his colleagues at the Permanente Medical Group in Oakland, California. I wrote 450 questions about family, personal, and social history as well as what physicians call a "review of systems," which consisted of questions about anatomical regions, such as bones, joints, and muscles, as well as problems with the respiratory, cardiovascular, gastrointestinal, genitourinary, and nervous systems. The questions were presented to each patient on a printed Hollerith card, which was punched with the code of the question. The patient responded by placing the card in a tray labeled either "yes," "no," "don't know," or "don't understand." The patient was then asked to qualify each problem, as indicated by its card in the "yes" tray, by taking an accompanying set of cards, with questions about onset, frequency, duration, and severity, and placing each card into its appropriately labeled tray. The sorted cards were then fed to a computer (a Control Data 1604 machine), where a program written by Lawrence Van Cura processed the results and generated a printed summary, in a legible but otherwise traditional format.

We interviewed thirty-seven patients with this system. All were receiving radiation therapy for cancer and had complicated histories. The card sorting turned out to be tiring and lengthy (over two hours), and only seventeen patients were able to finish because of scheduling dilemmas and time limitations beyond their control. Even though our patients' reaction to the program was generally favorable, we needed a better way to obtain a detailed medical history. It had occurred to me that a computer might actually *conduct* the medical interview, but I knew of no machine that was up to the job.

ENTER THE LINC

It was Philip Hicks who offered the solution. He suggested that we use the LINC (laboratory instrument computer) to take a medical history. He was already using the LINC to develop his programs, the first of their kind, for use in the clinical laboratories at the University of Wisconsin Hospitals. This small, general-purpose digital computer was developed at the Massachusetts Institute of Technology in 1962 by Wesley Clark, Charles Molnar, and their colleagues; it was a pioneering machine, and in many respects was the forerunner of today's personal computers. Flexibility and ease of operation were stressed in the development of the LINC. With it, the individual user could exert maximum control over the computer—a major departure from the batch-processing brontosaurs of the day. Designed to interact with the environment, the LINC was equipped with relays, sense switches, sense lines, analog-to-digital conversion channels (converting electronic signals such as wave forms to numbers), toggle switches, a cathode-ray oscilloscope that could double as a display screen, a typewriter keyboard, and a teletype printer.

Thus the LINC was well suited for *on-line* collection (that is, collection of data directly by the computer) and *real-time* processing (processing data as fast as they are generated). It found widespread use in neurophysiology laboratories, where it could be programmed to study the electrical activity of the nervous system—to initiate stimuli, receive responses, and then alter subsequent stimuli contingent upon the nature of the responses received. This was a hands-on computer; the wires were all hanging out, so to speak. There were no computing committees or subcommittees, no director of computing or chief information officer, no Mr. Binary telling you to keep out or not to touch. Users loved it!

Philip and I hypothesized that we could program the LINC to communicate directly with the patient by means of questions, explanations, requests, and comments displayed on the cathode-ray screen. The patient, in turn, could communicate with the computer by means of the typewriter keyboard. The LINC had a very small memory by today's standards—1,024 twelve-bit words—barely enough to hold the text for one question, together with the instructions in the program that told the computer what to do. The off-the-shelf personal computer of today is likely to bring with it about sixty-four million bytes of memory—about thirty-two thousand times as much memory as the LINC. The memory wasn't a crippling limitation, however—two magnetic tape drives, which could turn equally well in either direction, provided storage space for additional text and instructions that could quickly be called into memory when needed.

The LINC was also slow by today's standards, and the time between iterative instructions that told the computer to display a character on the screen—time in which the computer was executing other instructions, such as commands to display other characters—resulted in a flicker that became increasingly noticeable as the number of characters increased. There was reason, therefore, to keep the questions short, and this electronically imposed succinctness had a beneficial effect on the quality of my writing.

BEGINNINGS OF PATIENT-COMPUTER DIALOGUE

In addition to our practical concerns, my colleagues and I were motivated by a theoretical question: Could a computer be programmed to model the clinician as an interviewer? Could it actually interview a patient?

Our idea was to incorporate into the computer program at least some of the advantages of the physician as an interviewer: the ability to explore abnormal findings in detail and to personalize the interview in an appropriate, dignified, and considerate manner. At the same time, we wanted to gain the advantages of the questionnaire: its completeness, standardization, and, if possible, low cost.

We hoped that the computer-based interview would be helpful to the doctor in the care of the patient, that using the computer would be of interest to the patient (perhaps even enjoyable), and that pooled responses from many interviews would help us to learn more about the importance of the questions in the interview and to study the process of clinical interviewing. In addition to thinking about using computers in hospitals, clinics, and physicians' offices, I had the idea of a "medical history mobile," similar to the chest X-ray mobile of the era, that would serve prospective patients in remote parts of our country. And in the back of my mind was the idea that perhaps the computer could actually help patients to help themselves with medical problems.

Some of our colleagues considered the idea radical. Those who questioned the use of the computer in medicine under any circumstances were particularly concerned about the use of a machine to take a medical history—a time-honored traditional interaction between doctor and patient, hallowed ground in Western medicine. Some said it could not be done; others wondered if it *should* be done. Still others said that patients would find the idea offensive and would refuse to be interviewed by a computer, regardless of the nature of the program. (Years later, in completion of the critic's circle, they would ask, "Isn't everybody doing it?")

Patients, however, were remarkably enthusiastic. "It sounds like fun" and "I'd like to try my hand with a computer" were typical responses, particularly if (as was most often the case in 1965) they had never seen a computer. Their one concern was that the computer might try to perform an "intelligence test"—they didn't like intelligence tests. I assured them that I didn't either, and that I didn't even believe in what psychometricians call "intelligence tests." If anything, I wanted our computer to *do away* with these tests. They liked the idea and seemed relieved.

Starting with "A," I picked allergies for our first computer-based history. This seemed like a neutral, inoffensive subject for a computer; it is a field of great medical importance that relies heavily on the medical history, and our allergist consultant, Charles Reed, gave his enthusiastic support. We also mistakenly thought that an allergy history would be short. By the time we called a halt to expansion there were over five hundred questions in the program.

We used one of the original LINCs, which had been brought to the University of Wisconsin's neurophysiology laboratory by Joseph Hind. The machine was in great demand, and programming time during the day was scarce; we did most of our work between 10 P.M. and 8 A.M. Within a few months we had the program written and working well, but found ourselves continuing to make revisions. Most of these were minor and, in retrospect, inconsequential, and eventually I had to own up to the fact that I was procrastinating. It had been fun to talk about a computer that could take a medical history, to shock the traditionalists, and to argue with the skeptics, but to try it with a real patient— *for the first time*—that was another matter.

The First Patient

The time came, however, when I decided it was now or never. I approached one of our medical interns and asked him if he could select a patient for me. He seemed amused by the idea; he was tired— he had been up all night, as part of the draconian tradition in American medicine that doctors in training should go without sleep—and the thought of being replaced by a computer, at least at night, had a distinct appeal. He suggested a patient who might be willing to help, an elderly man who was recovering from a heart attack and was now up and about, getting ready to go home. I went to his room, introduced myself, told him the general idea of the project, explained that I didn't know how well it would work, and asked if he would give us a hand. "I'll try anything once," he replied, and he walked with me to the medical sciences building, where the LINC was housed. Fortunately, there was a free hour at lunchtime for us to try our first interview. Game as he was, I couldn't have expected our volunteer to visit the computer at 2 A.M. I turned on the machine, spun in the program from tape, turned off the lights in the room (the dim characters on the screen were easier to read in the dark), pressed the start button, and stepped back to observe.

This was not a randomized, controlled, double-blind experiment suitable for statistical analysis. It was more like cultural anthropology. In the tradition of Margaret Mead, I had put a machine in the clinical village, and stood by as unobtrusively as possible to see what would happen. Werner Heisenberg once noted that in science, the process of observation itself tends to influence the variables under scrutiny and thereby influence the findings. He derived his famous Uncertainty Principle from observations in physics, but the problem of uncertainty is nowhere more apparent than in the social sciences. The psychologist in the inner city, the criminologist in the federal prison, the anthropologist in the Third World village, and I in the LINC room, by our very presence, tend to affect the activities we hope to examine, and thus stand to compromise our own results. But in this instance, in the LINC room, my volunteer seemed truly oblivious to my presence.

The tapes churned, and "HAVE YOU EVER HAD HIVES?" appeared on the screen. The characters flickered, the lights on the console flashed on and off, and the LINC's speaker emitted an eerie, high-pitched sound. We had the computer, but its owners on the other side were still doing a cat brain experiment. On the other side of the sheetrock partition, people were walking in and out, and a cat was meowing. It was somewhat like Kafka's *Castle* or Koestler's *Darkness at Noon*.

Yet my newfound friend seemed oblivious to his surroundings. He got going at the keyboard, responding appropriately to the questions, and after a while it became clear that there was rapport between man and machine. He laughed out loud at some of the comments from the computer. Some I had intended to be funny; some I hadn't. And he talked to the machine, sometimes in praise and sometimes in criticism. "You already asked me that question," he noted with a taunting laugh. He was right, of course, although I rationalized that we could use the results, psychometrically, to check for test-retest reliability. He never would have criticized me face to face, a doctor with a white coat and a Bakelite nametag.

For most patients, even today, the doctor presents an authoritarian figure. By contrast, the computer did not seem at all authoritarian to this man; he was comfortable with it and felt free to be frank, even critical. Here was patient power at work. At the conclusion of the interview, he turned to me and said, "You know, I really like your computer better than some of those doctors over in the hospital."

Surprised, I asked him why.

"Well, for one thing, I'm sort of deaf and have trouble hearing them," he answered.

The Patient's Chart Declassified

For each of the possible responses to the computer's questions, we had developed phrases that could be printed when applicable. To appease those colleagues who clung to professional mystique, we converted words such as *hives* and *hay fever* to *urticaria* and *allergic rhinitis*. The computer was programmed to print these phrases, as with our card sorting program, in a legible but otherwise traditional format for use by the doctor.

When our first patient had completed his interview, I was relieved to hear the Teletype chatter as it began to print; the summary program was working. He then turned to me and said, "What's happening? May I read that?" I could not think of any reason why he shouldn't. Once again, the computer was helping him to assert himself as a patient.

This may have been the first time that a patient at the University of Wisconsin Hospitals was offered the opportunity to read his own record. As he started to read, he commented suddenly, in reference to some details about his hay fever: "No, that's wrong; I didn't mean that," and he then proceeded to pick out other errors. Clearly, there were mistakes in the interview. Yet if he hadn't asked to read his summary, I might never have known.

We learned our lesson, and since that time have asked our patients, whenever they are willing, to read their summaries, help us edit their medical histories, and thereby improve our computer-based interviews. And patients' criticisms have been most helpful over the years. Whether we are writing at a keyboard or in longhand, it is unrealistic and often demeaning for us to record our interpretation of what patients tell us without letting them see what we've written, and when doctors do so they may perpetuate errors that could be corrected. Furthermore, there is a natural tendency to find fault with the patient when difficulties arise; diagnoses such as "inadequate personality" would have disappeared quickly if patients had seen them early on. I realized that for patients who want to be active participants in their medical care, the medical record should be declassified for them as quickly as possible. I looked forward to the time when the medical chart, traditionally closed to the patient, would become a document developed jointly by patient and doctor.

A Formal Study

Encouraged by the results of this first interview, we did a more formal study. Fifty hospitalized patients agreed to have their allergy histories taken. In each case, we compared the results of the computer's history as printed out on the Teletype with the allergy history as recorded in the hospital chart by the medical student, intern, resident, and staff physician who were caring for the patient.

In medical parlance, because of the traditional orientation to disease rather than health, a *positive* finding denotes the presence of a disease and a *negative* finding denotes its absence. The computer interview contained no "false negative findings"—that is, the computer identified all the allergies mentioned in the patients' charts.

Among patients whose charts gave no indication of allergies, the computer elicited two cases of asthma, seven cases of hay fever, twelve cases of hives, and one case of allergy to penicillin. In this instance, the medical student's workup did mention a rash in association with penicillin, but to find it one had to read the workup from beginning to end; the intern's note stated "no allergies." With another patient, the mention of "penicillin allergy" in the chart was insufficient to determine whether an allergy actually existed, whereas the computer described the single reaction in detail and left no doubt that a serious serum-sickness type of reaction had occurred and that this person should be advised never to take penicillin again. All adverse drug reactions were described in more detail by the computer than by the students and doctors.

On the other hand, the computer elicited and printed out several "false positive" findings, such as an "allergic reaction" to phenobarbital that the patient later described as "excessive grogginess," not an allergy.

At the end of the interview, the computer asked each patient what he or she had thought of the experience. As we had hoped, almost all the patients found their interaction with the computer both interesting and enjoyable. When asked to compare the computer interviews with interviews conducted by doctors, twenty patients had no preference, twelve indicated a preference for physician-taken histories, and—to our surprise—eighteen indicated a preference for the computer-based system. (Of course, if the doctor and not the computer had asked this question, the results might have been different.)

Further Studies in Madison and Boston

Heartened by these early results, we pressed on with further studies of computer-based medical interviews in our laboratory at the University of Wisconsin. We developed and studied histories for patients with problems such as cancer and epilepsy. The uterine cancer interview, which was written by Ben Peckham, his colleagues in the Department of Gynecology, Lawrence Van Cura, and me, asked questions about sexual activity, menstruation, pregnancies, bleeding, and past gynecological problems. Most patients indicated that they found their time at the computer to be both worthwhile and interesting, and that they had a slight preference for the computer as an interviewer in comparison with physicians in their experience. Once again, however, the computer was doing the asking.

The topics in this interview were of a sensitive, personal nature. It was particularly interesting to me, therefore, to hear from the women who had taken the interview, which was done in private, that they had sometimes been more comfortable while communicating information to the computer about potentially embarrassing matters such as sexual activity than they would have been while talking to their doctor. Even when they wanted the physician to receive the information, as would be the case when the doctor read the computer's printed summary, they found it easier to tell it to the machine. This observation, which we first reported in 1968, has since been corroborated in a number of studies in a variety of settings. The computer interview under some circumstances seems to facilitate a form of *abreaction,* or the verbal release of repressed information.

With the interview for patients with epilepsy, Raymond Chun and I compared the computer's printed summaries with the handwritten summaries of residents and staff physicians, and found that the computer's summaries contained more information about the patients' symptoms before, during, and after their seizures. Again, patients reacted favorably to the computer interview.

After coming to Boston, I continued my research with patient-computer dialogue at Harvard teaching hospitals. Our studies of computer interviews for patients with headache were directed by Alan Leviton and his colleagues Dhirendra Bana and John Graham from the Headache Research Foundation. In one study, forty patients who participated found the interview to be interesting, thoughtful, and considerate. Thirty-eight found the computer program easy to use, but only twenty-two thought that the computer had been complete in taking the history of their headaches. Clearly, additions and revisions were in order.

Six internists and one neurologist, each with a strong interest in headache studies, reviewed the printed summaries of these computer histories and incorporated them into their clinical evaluations. For twenty-two of their patients, the physicians indicated that the summaries had been helpful in their evaluations; for seven patients, the computer had clarified the nature of the headache, and for five patients, the computer had provided information that was not available in the personal history. In most instances, the physicians indicated that they would like to use the computer's summaries in the future.

When we analyzed patients' responses to the computer and compared them with physicians' diagnoses, we found that precursors of headaches, such as changes in vision, changes in weather, and consumption of alcohol, which are generally believed to be unique to the diagnosis of migraine, were almost as frequent among patients with muscle contraction or tension headache. We concluded that muscle contraction headache is more similar to migraine than is generally recognized.

When we were doing our studies back in the 1970s and 1980s, people rarely had access to a computer. It was gratifying, therefore, to discover that school-age children with no computer experience would respond enthusiastically to their time with the computer interview designed specifically for them—an interview that was able to elicit detailed information about their headaches. Interestingly, our findings indicated that doctors were reluctant—more so than they are today—to classify recurring headaches in children as migraine.

Also, first in Madison and then in Boston, we were working to develop a comprehensive computer-based general medical history—a complete history for all seasons and all situations. As a derivative of my card-sorting program, this started with a rudimentary review of body systems, such as the heart, lungs, and abdomen, branching to a few questions for qualification of each abnormality. Over the years, we have revised this history, made it more detailed in some areas and less detailed in others, and (in collaboration with Guerdon Coombs and Patricia Downs) modified it to the needs of individual clinics, such as the Marshfield Clinic in rural Wisconsin and the Harvard Street Clinic in Boston—where it was translated into French and Spanish to accommodate patients who had recently immigrated from Haiti and Puerto Rico.

We were also exploring yet additional roles for the computer as an interviewing machine. In 1968, John Greist and I developed an employment interview—a computer-based session for applicants to the medical internship program at the University of Wisconsin Hospital. The computer asked about each applicant's hopes and wants for an internship and then offered detailed information about the program in Madison. In a small experimental trial, applicants reacted favorably to the interview and felt that it was a valuable addition to their visit to the hospital.

SPREADING THE WORD

In the meantime, others began to work in the field. A general medical history, with emphasis on the review of systems, was developed and studied by John Mayne and his colleagues at the Mayo Clinic, and both patients and physicians reacted favorably. The computer obtained 95 percent of the information about the symptoms that had been recorded in the traditional medical record. Another general medical history was studied by Jerome Grossman and his colleagues at the Massachusetts General Hospital, where patients also reacted favorably. Physicians' attitudes were mixed, but the computer's summaries were in good agreement with the physicians' findings. A general medical history was also studied at LDS Hospital in Salt Lake City by Homer Warner and his colleagues. With this history, Bayes's theorem—a mathematical technique to estimate the likelihood of different outcomes—was used to make diagnostic suggestions on the basis of patients' responses to the computer. Meanwhile, other investigators were developing and evaluating histories in a wide variety of medical areas, such as allergy, emergency room medicine, gastrointestinal problems, general health assessment, headache, nutrition, and venereal disease. Research in the field of computer-based interviewing remains active to this day. Patient-computer dialogue is not as yet readily available in most clinical settings, but I am optimistic that it will be in the not-too-distant future.

The Patient in Control

The idea of a computer taking a medical history can evoke worrisome thoughts: *2001: A Space Odyssey, Terminal Man, Invasion of the Body Snatchers,* Orwellian thought control. Yet the experience of our first patient—as with the majority of patients who have subsequently engaged in dialogue with our computers—was the opposite of what some had predicted. This man had *gained* control, not lost it. For the first time in his role as a patient, *he* was in charge; he was master of his own history. And in his world of deafness he could communicate particularly well with the machine.

THE MECHANICS OF THE INTERVIEW

The power of the computer as an interviewing machine is in its *branching*, that is, moving from frame (or display) to frame in a manner contingent on the patient's responses. In this way the computer can ask questions, answer questions in turn, teach the meaning of concepts not understood, give advice and suggestions, and provide words of encouragement, even with a bit of humor here and there. As I gained experience in writing interviews, I found myself better able to use this new medium to personalize the dialogue and transfer control from the computer to the person engaged in dialogue with the computer.

The Dialogue

Typically, the patient interacts with the computer by means of the screen and keyboard or mouse on a computer terminal, or more recently, on a personal computer or laptop. The computer communicates with the patient by means of text displayed on the screen, and the patient communicates with the computer by means of the keyboard or mouse. If a person is blind or illiterate, a surrogate can read the questions on the screen.

In several studies, a digitized human or computer-generated voice has presented the questions. Such techniques have promise, particularly when used in telephone interviews, as in the programs of Lee Baer and John Greist and their colleagues, because the telephone is more readily available than the personal computer. If the person is deaf, however, voice is unusable unless a surrogate is available to sign. Computers that can recognize the spoken word have great potential for the future, but for the present, they are not generally available— and in any case, most models today have limited vocabularies and imperfect accuracy, even after training for individual users.

With our programs, the dialogue between computer and patient usually begins with words of welcome. "Hello! It's good to be 'talking' with you today. To begin, please press the 'Enter' key on the keyboard." If the patient does so, the computer continues: "Exactly, pressing 'Enter' is the way to continue. Why not try it again?" And, if "Enter" is pressed again, the computer responds with "You have a nice touch with the keys." This typically elicits a bit of laughter, and the interview is under way.

The dialogue then continues with instruction on how to use the keyboard. The patient must be able to read the frames on the screen and be capable of sustained mental activity to interact with the computer during the introductory and teaching sections. If all goes well with these beginning frames, the patient is likely to be ready for the medical questions. If the patient cannot negotiate the opening sequences, personal intervention is warranted.

Over the years, we have incorporated into our programs a number of provisions designed to yield control to the patient in dialogue with the computer. With the typical interview, we request permission to proceed (for example, "May we call you by your first name?" and "Would it be OK with you if we asked a few questions about your emotions?"). We do our best to respect the patients' priorities, to respect their right to decide (with sufficient alternatives), *not* to decide, to help with uncertainty (offering "don't know" and "don't understand" options, with explanations when appropriate), and to respect reluctance to respond.

Communication between patient and computer—like that between patient and doctor—should not be used to persuade the patient to answer questions the doctor deems important; rather, it should be used to outline the medical reasons for the questions so that patients can decide for themselves whether they care to answer. Patients should not have to answer questions against their will. In Wisconsin, we incorporated a "none of your damn business" option into the questions. We have since toned it down to "skip it," better accepted in Boston.

An expanded set of responses to yes-no questions enables patients to indicate uncertainty and lack of comprehension, to request clarification, and to bypass questions they don't care to answer. This reduces the number of uninformed responses and the coercion that can lead to inconsistency, subterfuge, and decreased validity. Most of our computer-based interviews also employ, to some extent, other mutually exclusive numbered choices, multiple choices with more than one response acceptable, and free-text responses. We have also incorporated into our programs the ability to monitor automatically the time it takes a person to respond at the keyboard. The computer can then use this information, in addition to the person's keyboard responses, as a condition for determining the course of the interview. A prolonged response time, for example, which might indicate a patient's uncertainty when responding to a question, can be used as a condition for pursuing the subject further.

In our experience, and the experience of most others who have studied dialogue between patient and computer, concern about the computer as a depersonalizing influence in dialogue with patients has been unfounded. Most patients who have had the opportunity "to talk to the computer" have found their experience to be pleasant, interesting, and informative.

PATIENT POWER

In the spring of 1970, I discussed my ideas on patient power at a conference at the University of Michigan in Ann Arbor. Those in attendance were divided in their reaction, and the ensuing debate was heated. The moderator, John Romano (chair of the Department of Psychiatry at the University of Rochester), staunchly defended the right of the physician to direct the patient ("patients want to be told what to do"); Leonard Savage (professor of statistics at Yale), on the other hand, said that he "was particularly pleased to hear the bold and radical defense of the thesis that medical values should be those of the patient."

The debate was to continue through the 1970s. Franz Ingelfinger, editor of the *New England Journal of Medicine,* rejected my article "The Patient's Right to Decide," making it clear in his letter that he strongly disagreed with my position. On the other hand, Ian Monroe, editor of the *Lancet* (to whom I will be forever grateful), sent me an encouraging letter of acceptance and published my article forthwith. But all agreed during those decades of debate that when it came to dialogue between patient and computer, the patient should be in charge. Ironically, transferring control to the patient was more readily accomplished by means of an automaton than by means of the physician.

The next step in our studies of patient-computer dialogue was to move beyond programs that take the medical history, which were designed primarily to collect information from the patient for use by the doctor. Our idea was to use the computer as a *patient's* assistant—to develop interactive computer programs that would help patients help themselves, as well as help their doctors.

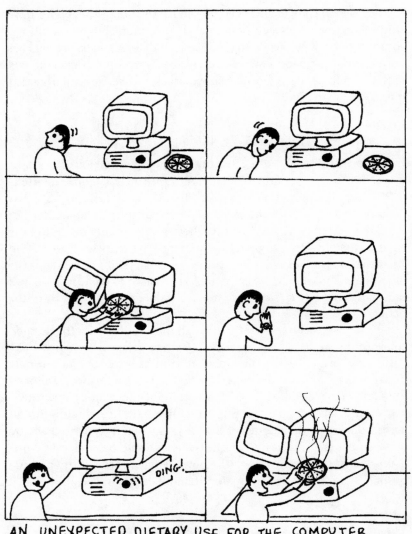

AN UNEXPECTED DIETARY USE FOR THE COMPUTER

CHAPTER THREE

Cybermedicine as a Patient's Assistant

O ur early studies of dialogue between patient and computer were based on the premise that the computer interview could be helpful to the doctor for purposes of diagnosis and treatment. The next step was to develop programs that would be helpful to the *patient* in diagnosis and treatment.

GUIDELINES FOR A PATIENT'S PROGRAM

In developing interactive programs for patients, I have tried to keep these guidelines in mind:

- *The program should be medically sound.* The authors' credentials and relevant experience should be readily available for scrutiny.

- *The program should be easy to use.* It should be designed by people who understand the psychology of conversation with a computer, the human factors as well as the medical content. A few keystrokes or clicks of the mouse should be sufficient to gain access to the program, and moving from the opening words of welcome to the various options within the program should be straightforward. Ideally, the program should be addressed to the literacy level of the user, and written in the user's native language.

- *The program should be truly interactive.* Obtaining information from the computer should be easier than from a pamphlet or book. The program should be more than a page turner; the opposable thumb and forefinger are quite sufficient for this on their own, without benefit of electronics. The program should respond quickly to the wishes and needs of the individual user. It should also proffer appropriate and potentially useful alternatives that the person has not yet thought of. It should ask questions with respect and thoughtfulness and answer questions in the same manner. When called upon to do so, the program should offer explanations, instructions, and suggestions.

- *The program should be of immediate benefit to the user.* The emphasis should be on the practical. Theoretical underpinnings and background information should be available to those who want to pursue them, but strategies for dealing with the situation at hand must be available first and foremost—at the top of the electronic menu, so to speak. A user might want to know the biochemistry of clotting blood, but not while coping with a bleeding cut.

- *The patient should be in charge.* The patient's right to respond or not to respond, to decide or not to decide, should be honored. When reluctance to respond or to decide is due to lack of information or confusion, the program should inform or clarify. Further, the program should respect the patient's priorities by offering choices during the course of the interview and by requesting permission to proceed.

- *Confidentiality should be protected.* Only the individual user or persons whom the user has authorized should have access to the information obtained during the dialogue. The capability should exist, however, for pooling data from consenting users, who would remain anonymous, for use both in improving the program and in clinical research.

- *The program should be readily available.* People of all socioeconomic backgrounds should be able to use it in a place of convenience and at an affordable cost. Access to the computer should be as easy as access to the telephone.

- *The computer should be fast and reliable.* In the event of problems, help should be on hand.

- *The program should be subjected to formal study with volunteers in an experimental setting, before being offered to the public.* Results of the study, including helpfulness of the program, safety, and satisfaction of the volunteers, should be available to all who might subsequently want to use the program.

To my knowledge, no program yet exists that achieves this ideal. Certainly none of ours do. On the other hand, a number of people in the field are making progress, and I am optimistic.

—◦◦◦—

In our laboratory, Howard Bleich, Hollis Kowaloff, Alan Leviton, Steven Locke, Douglas Porter, Charles Safran, Jelia Witschi, our colleagues, and I have studied the interactive computer as a patient's assistant in a variety of health-related areas.

HELPING WITH WHAT WE EAT

We all have to eat and most of us would like to eat carefully but not to the point of compromising taste. Most of us know that some vitamins and minerals are essential and must be included in our diets. Most of us know that chronic, excessive consumption of carbohydrates can lead to overweight, and that dietary fat can make us more vulnerable to heart disease as we get older.

On the other hand, most of us will never be professional nutritionists, and we find ourselves these days confronted with a bewildering plethora of information in the press, often of a conflicting nature. It isn't just any fat that is bad for us, we read; saturated fat is the principal culprit. But knowing this we are still faced with questions such as which cooking oil to use (current wisdom favors olive oil) and which margarine to use in lieu of butter. Eating more calcium may be as important as eating less sodium to reduce blood pressure. Beta-carotene, once advocated as a vitamin supplement to help prevent cancer, has recently been declared ineffective. Caffeine keeps getting blamed as a causative substance for cancers such as cancer of the pancreas—and then exonerated. Although a diet high in refined carbohydrates such as the "simple" sugar sucrose is a causative factor in dental cavities in children, with fluoride in our drinking water, cavities have been reduced dramatically, independent of the amount of sugar we eat. Whether simple sugar is bad for us in other ways remains controversial.

In keeping with the state of confusion about nutrition and diet and our interest in the computer as a patient's assistant, my colleagues and I asked ourselves whether an interactive program might help people alter their dietary behavior, when indicated, to their nutritional advantage. This was really a rhetorical question; the answer in our minds was yes, and we set out to prove we were right. (There is no such person as a truly disinterested scientist.)

We proceeded to develop a dietary counseling interview in collaboration with Jelia Witschi of the Harvard School of Public Health, who became the mentor of the project. Writing in our programming language Converse (which we use for all our interviewing programs), we created an interview that would ask questions dealing with general dietary behavior, elicit details of food intake on an average day, and plan with a person a weight-reducing diet of approximately 1500 kcal. During the interview, the program would offer dietary suggestions and, on completion, generate a printed summary for use by patients and nutritionists.

An Experiment

In a study with sixty-four volunteers (thirty-two men and thirty-two women), each with the self-diagnosis of simple overweight, the interview was found to assist the patients in organizing their thoughts about eating and in planning their own dietary behavior, and also to assist the expert nutritionists participating in the study when they subsequently met with the volunteers. In addition, the patients found their time with the computer to be a pleasant and personalizing experience.

Fifty-six of the sixty-four patients returned for the three-month visit, which was scheduled as part of the study. Of these, thirty-six (64 percent) had lost an average of seven pounds; seven (13 percent) had no weight change; and thirteen (23 percent) had gained an average of five pounds.

It was not our intention to suggest that the weight loss in this experiment should be attributed to use of the computer. All volunteers had sessions with a nutritionist as well as the computer. However, we are confident that the conversational computer can be helpful in studying the relative effectiveness of various approaches to dialogue with people who want to lose weight, and we are equally confident that the computer will prove to be a good medium for such dialogue when an effective approach is found.

The computer interview was especially good at helping people understand their own thoughts and actions. Comments such as "It heightened awareness of eating habits"; "It gave me an almost exact picture of what I eat and drink daily"; and "The computer is your-self—you don't feel responsible to anyone except yourself" illustrate how useful participants found the process.

These comments suggest a personalizing effect that can be a par-ticular advantage of the computer as an interviewer. Conversation with a computer is, after all, similar in some ways to conversation with oneself. Soliloquy can sometimes be helpful in promoting insight and, at least in this experiment, the computer was successful in enhancing self-awareness.

The computer was better at asking questions than at answering them. Volunteers could indicate when they didn't understand or were uncertain about their answers, but there was little opportunity for them to query the machine directly. Accordingly, the experiment gave us valuable insight about how we could make our programs more responsive to people's needs.

A revised and updated version of this program is currently in rou-tine use by personnel at Beth Israel Deaconess Medical Center in Boston.

A PROGRAM FOR EMPLOYEE HEALTH

In 1985, Beth Israel Hospital, a major teaching hospital of Harvard Medical School, implemented Johnson and Johnson's "Live for Life" program. This voluntary program, which was designed to promote physical and emotional well-being among the hospital's personnel, consisted of a self-administered (pencil-and-paper) health question-naire, health education classes, and an exercise fitness center.

In 1990, in collaboration with clinicians at the hospital and mem-bers of the employee health department, we replaced the paper ques-tionnaire with a computer-administered health screening interview for hospital employees and staff clinicians. The interview then became part of the integrated Center for Clinical Computing (CCC) cyber-medicine system on an increasing number of terminals throughout the Beth Israel Hospital. Since 1998, subsequent to the merger of Beth

Israel and Deaconess hospitals in 1996 to form Beth Israel Deaconess Medical Center, the program has been available to approximately six thousand employees on more than eight thousand terminals located throughout the medical center. Conducted in private and with protection of confidentiality, the interview seeks information on medical problems and patterns of living for which behavioral change is considered desirable. It also offers advice and suggestions on matters of health and illness.

The Effect of Lifestyle

Like all our programs, the interview begins with words of welcome, information on how to proceed, and a brief discussion of the purpose of the program. ("We hope we can help you discover how your lifestyle affects your health and what you can do to improve your health.") It assures the user that all responses will be kept in confidence and made available to clinicians only at the user's request.

Next there is a series of frames that teach the inexperienced user how to operate the computer terminal, how to change answers and back up to previous questions, and how to indicate uncertainty—by choosing "don't understand" or "maybe (don't know)"—and reluctance to respond—by choosing "skip it."

The interview itself begins with a section that elicits demographic information, with emphasis on the circumstances of each participant's employment at the hospital. The computer then lists the seven sections of the interview (General Medical History, Nutrition History, Exercise Patterns, Habits, Safety, Environment, and Stress) and offers participants the opportunity to select sections in the order of their personal preference.

An optional component of the nutrition section is the twenty-four-hour recall, which begins by identifying the first meal or snack of the day and then asks about six potential eating periods. When the user has responded to all questions about a specific meal or snack, the program provides a chance to check the accuracy of the entries and list additional foods that come to mind. At the conclusion of the nutrition section, the user is asked to evaluate the accuracy and completeness of the entries and to indicate whether the meals or foods listed reflect typical eating patterns; if not, the program asks in what ways they are unusual. The twenty-four-hour recall may be repeated as often as desired.

As each section is completed, the program offers to display a summary of the information provided. With the nutrition section, the summary details the specific nutrients in each food eaten, with totals for each meal and total nutrient intake for the day plus a dietary evaluation showing actual and recommended nutrients.

At the end of the interview, the program offers a clinical evaluation of problems elicited by the interview that could be favorably influenced by changes in behavior. In addition, the program offers information about referral services. If, for example, a person mentions feeling depressed, the program provides the names and telephone numbers of places to turn to for help—the Employee Assistance Program, the Samaritans, and the hospital's emergency room.

Use of the Program

Over the past ten years, 3,335 employees have completed the interview. Each interview took about thirty minutes from start to finish. Most of the participants (97 percent) were between twenty and sixty years of age. About half of them referred to themselves as "professional" (nurses are the largest group of employees), and the rest as "clerical or secretarial," "technical," "managerial," or "service" workers; 1 percent preferred not to answer this question.

During the course of the interview, 85 percent of the employees expressed an interest in the health-related programs offered by the hospital: 73 percent were interested in the fitness center, 38 percent in the stress-reduction program, 24 percent in the "management of your time" program, 12 percent in the low-back protection program, and 6 percent in the smoking-cessation program.

Thirty-two percent of the participants who completed the interview availed themselves of the opportunity to visit the nurse for a follow-up evaluation and to consider entering one or more of the health-related programs. Fourteen percent answered yes to the question "Would you like to get more information about [safe sex practices] when you visit with the nurse?" Nine percent answered yes when asked "Do you have any questions about birth control?"—and most of these answered yes to the question "Would you like to talk about this when you visit with the nurse?" When participants communicated a desire to be contacted directly for further information and recommendations, this was forwarded to the nurse. With future versions of the program, we would like the computer program itself to be equipped to provide this information directly to those employees who would like it, on-line.

More than half the employees at the hospital who took the health screening interview also took the computerized twenty-four-hour dietary recall, and almost a third took it more than once. It was gratifying to learn from these people that the program was helping them to alter their diets in accordance with current nutritional wisdom as well as in a beneficial manner, from their personal perspective.

Real and potential difficulties in life are common among hospital personnel, as indicated by the results of the interview: 57 percent of the respondents reported high levels of stress, and 43 percent reported feeling sad, discouraged, or hopeless in the previous month; 6 percent indicated that life sometimes did not seem worth living. (As soon as their responses were registered, these people were told by the computer where they could obtain help for their problems.) We hope these employees moved quickly to avail themselves of the opportunity offered by the computer.

As we have found with other computer-based interviews, the participants reacted favorably to this one: 85 percent responded positively when asked whether their time at the computer was worthwhile. The participants who indicated that they wanted to pursue health-related matters further were more likely to have found the interview worthwhile. The interview, it would seem, served to facilitate an interest in health and well-being.

When asked to compare the computer-based interview with an interview with a doctor or nurse, more participants indicated a preference for the computer. As in our earlier studies, however, the computer posed this question. Had a nurse or doctor asked the same question, the answer might have been different.

Sixteen percent of the participants answered yes when asked, "Did the computer sometimes ask you more than you wanted to tell?" By contrast, 50 percent answered yes to "Did you sometimes want to tell the computer more than it asked?" Furthermore, participants were more likely to find the interview worthwhile if they were among those who wanted to tell the computer more than it asked. We interpreted these results as an indication that we were on the right track and that we should expand the program to make it more receptive and more informative.

Times are difficult for many people in this country, as reflected by the findings in our study. Personnel in hospitals and clinics, whose mission is to minister to the needs of others, often suffer undue physical and emotional hardships of their own—both at work and in their private lives. The health-promotion programs of the Beth Israel Deaconess Medical Center are offered to all hospital personnel, with the hope that people will become active participants in their own care. And people are using the programs every day. We hope other hospitals will do what Beth Israel Deaconess Medical Center is doing to promote well-being among their own employees.

SELF-CARE

Urinary tract infection is a common and important medical problem among women, from adolescence through later life. By contrast, it is rare among men under the age of fifty. The anatomical reason for this disparity is the difference in the length of the urethra, the tube from the bladder through which urine is excreted. Being shorter in women, the urethra is less of a protective barrier to bacteria, which can find their way into the bladder and (in a culture of residual urine) initiate a cystitis, or infection of the bladder. If the bacteria should then ascend to a kidney through one of the connecting ureters, a more serious kidney infection, or pyelonephritis, can result. In the great majority of cases, however, the infection remains in the bladder, an "uncomplicated urinary tract infection" that is readily cured—in most instances with one of the sulfa drugs.

Urinary tract infections treated in the traditional manner require individualized attention by a physician or nurse practitioner in a clinical setting—professional care that is inconvenient for the patient, sometimes unavailable, and always expensive. In the United States, urinary tract infections result in over six million visits to doctors' offices or other medical facilities each year. With a conservative estimate of $50 per visit, not including the cost of laboratory studies and medication, this is an annual expenditure of $300 million.

Consequently, my colleagues and I hypothesized that as an alternative, patient-computer dialogue could provide the basis for the diagnosis and treatment of urinary tract infections in a manner at least as good as an office visit. We further hypothesized that this automated patient's assistant could be made available in the home, school, or workplace, in a manner substantially less expensive than traditional professional care. And we hoped that principles derived from a study with urinary tract infection could be applied to the computer as an assistant to patients with other common, important medical problems.

The Patient's Assistant

In perhaps our most radical departure from the traditional, Howard Bleich, Linda Fisher, Scott Johnson, Douglas Porter, and I set about to test our hypothesis. In 1975, we developed a program designed to assist women in caring for themselves when suffering from an uncomplicated urinary tract infection. Integrated into the program were questions designed to make certain that the woman's infection was in fact uncomplicated; any indication of a more serious problem, for example, a history of fever that might indicate a kidney infection, would result in the recommendation that the patient seek further medical care from a physician. The program was designed for experimental trial in a clinical setting with close medical supervision by doctors and nurses. The long-range goal, however, was to have this program, if successful, modified for use by patients in their homes.

The Experimental Program

The program begins with the usual words of welcome and a sequence of instructions about how to take the interview. It then takes a history of the symptoms usually associated with a urinary tract infection. ("If it is OK with you, we would now like to ask a few questions about urinary symptoms." Consent is followed by, "Are you bothered by pain or burning when you urinate?" "Are you urinating more often than you usually do?" and "Are you bothered by the unexpected, urgent need to urinate?")

The program then offers the patient instructions about providing a urine sample for analysis (to check for white blood cells, which might indicate an infection) and culture (to identify any bacteria that might be causing an infection). The interview is interrupted to allow the patient to provide a urine sample for laboratory studies. When the patient returns, the program resumes with medical questions dealing with urinary, gynecological, cardiological, gastrointestinal, and metabolic problems (for example, "Have you felt feverish within the past few days?" and "Have you ever been told by a doctor that you have high blood pressure?") to rule out complicating problems that would need care beyond the scope of the program. The program also tests the reliability of important questions by repeating them, and it resolves uncertainties that may arise, for example, when the patient does not understand a question. In the event of an abnormality or possible abnormality that might preclude continued participation, the medical logic incorporated into the program is used to construct words of advice and explanation and to suggest that the patient meet with a doctor.

If the program detects no reasons for referral, including no history of untoward experiences with sulfa, it proceeds to the therapy section, which presents six topics of possible concern about medication— effectiveness, cost, safety, dosage, route of administration, and "Can I get well without it?"—discusses these as they relate to treatment with sulfa, in the order of importance chosen by the patient—"You indicated that knowing how well sulfa works is perhaps most important to you. Let's consider this first"—and offers opportunities to review information previously presented—"Before deciding about sulfa, would you like to go over anything again?"

Deciding for Yourself

Thereby informed, the patient is offered the choice of taking sulfa, taking nothing, considering another medicine, or indicating uncertainty. If the time to respond to this question is particularly long or short compared with a previous more neutral question (the program keeps track of response time automatically), the program mentions this and asks if the patient would like to reconsider her choice. (Short response times may indicate confident decision or uninformed consent; long response times may indicate thoughtful weighing of alternatives or considerable doubt.)

As a further check for reliability, the patient is asked to indicate her decision at least twice. Patients who elect not to take sulfa are offered referral to a doctor. Those who elect to take sulfa are offered the option to start it immediately or to wait for the results of the culture. For those who elect to begin sulfa right away, the computer provides a suggested medication schedule. The program concludes with a series of questions about the patient's reaction to the interview—whether the program was helpful and whether she liked deciding for herself about taking the medicine.

The computer then prints out for the patient her medication schedule, a summary of the interview, a list of the signs of an adverse reaction to the sulfa, and a prescription to be filled in the pharmacy of her choice. The patient is then asked to call our laboratory at once if she is feeling worse or has reacted adversely to the sulfa, and to call in any event after three or four days to get the results of her culture and further advice.

Follow-Up

A research assistant receives the follow-up telephone calls and enters the patient's responses to a detailed computer interview, which is read to the patient, at the computer terminal. With structured questions and suggestions presented by the computer, the assistant asks the patient whether her symptoms have disappeared, whether she has been able to take the medicine, and whether she has had any other problems.

Rules incorporated into the logic of the program guide the assistant in advising the patient over the phone and scheduling a return visit. If symptoms are persistent or there is evidence of a possible adverse reaction to the medication, the patient is advised to stop all medication and to return to the clinic as soon as possible. If the symptoms have abated, the patient is advised to return to the clinic in two weeks and, if she is willing, an appointment is scheduled. Patients who do not call within four days are contacted by the research assistant for the telephone interview.

A patient who returns for the follow-up visit is interviewed by the computer about urinary symptoms, whether she was able to take the medicine, and any problems that might have arisen. Then, after a brief review of instructions by the computer, she is asked to provide another urine sample for a repeat analysis and culture. If the interview or urinalysis indicates a persistent or recurrent infection, or if new symptoms require attention, the patient is referred by the computer to a physician. If the repeat urine culture demonstrates infecting bacteria, the patient is called and advised to return for further evaluation and treatment.

Putting the Program to the Test

In a preliminary clinical trial, the program performed to the satisfaction of the patients who participated and those of us who designed the study. Of forty-six patients who came to the clinic for help with their symptoms, which included pain with urination, ten were referred out of the program for consultation with a doctor, and thirty-six continued on to the therapy section of the interview. Among the thirty-six women who completed the program, "How well does the medicine work?" "Can I get well without it?" and "How safe is it?" were the most important considerations. Thirty-four of the patients decided to take the sulfa immediately, one patient decided to wait for the results of her culture (which turned out to be negative), and one was uncertain, but later in the interview decided to take the sulfa.

Of the thirty-six patients who completed the interview, nineteen called our laboratory for their telephone interview, six were reached by one of us, and eleven could not be reached by telephone and were lost to the study. Of the twenty-five patients who were interviewed by telephone, twenty-four had taken at least some of their medicine, and the one who had not was about to start. Sixteen were asymptomatic and doing well, seven were feeling better, and two had not improved and were later lost to further follow-up.

Fourteen of the patients returned to our laboratory for their follow-up visit. Eleven were asymptomatic and three still had symptoms. On repeat culture, two of the asymptomatic patients and the three symptomatic patients had persistent bacterial infections and were referred to a doctor for further care. The volunteers in this study were not billed for their visits.

The return rate among the volunteers was low—only fourteen of thirty-six patients (39 percent) returned for their second visit. On the other hand, this compared favorably with the return rate of all our patients with urinary tract infections, which was in the range of 25 to 30 percent. (Note that the currently recommended three-day treatment of uncomplicated urinary tract infection—with a tablet containing sulfamethoxazole and trimethoprim—is so effective that follow-up appointments are for the most part no longer recommended.)

Of the forty-two patients who were asked about their reaction to the initial interview (four of the ten who were referred to a doctor were inadvertently not asked these questions) forty found the computer "considerate," thirty-eight found the computer "thoughtful" and "respectful," and thirty-eight found their time at the computer well spent. When the thirty-six patients who continued into the treatment section were asked "How has it been to decide for yourself about sulfa?" thirty found it to be "a good thing," three had "no preference either way," two were "not sure," and one thought it would be "better left up to someone else."

Upon leaving the session, patients spoke approvingly of their time with the computer: "No doctor has ever been as thorough with me as your machine" and "I hope you will have similar programs for other medical problems" were among the comments. And the majority of patients liked being able to make their own decisions about treatment.

This is consistent with all our findings on patient-computer dialogue. Concern about the computer as a depersonalizing influence in dialogue with patients has been unfounded. The interaction has been pleasant, interesting, informative, and empowering for the overwhelming majority of patients.

THE ISSUE OF COMPLIANCE

Physicians often complain that patients are noncompliant; they do not do what they are told. This resistance perplexes doctors. They can write prescriptions for patients, but they cannot control what patients do with the prescriptions.

I think it would be more appropriate to focus on the problem that may underlie noncompliance, the assumption that physicians are in charge of "their" patients and entitled to make decisions on their behalf. The very word *compliance* suggests submission to a higher authority.

I believe that patients who want to should be encouraged to make their own clinical decisions, as in our study of urinary tract infection, and that noncompliance should be regarded simply as disagreement with the doctor. Our data indicate that patients who elect to make their own medical decisions will be faithful to them, that they will do what they *tell themselves* to do. This has also been demonstrated by John Wennberg, Albert Mulley, and their colleagues when working with patients with diseases of the prostate gland. Furthermore, patients who make their own decisions will be responsible for the consequences of their choices, and their physicians will be spared the liability that accompanies medical paternalism. Self-reliant patients will be more realistic in their clinical expectations than patients who depend on their doctors' "orders." Subservient patients tend to regard their physicians as omniscient and are often incredulous when outcomes are unfavorable. As George Bernard Shaw pointed out years ago, this tendency may help explain why patients have been quick to sue and why doctors have fared poorly in court.

GOALS FOR THE FUTURE

Urinary tract infection is a medical problem traditionally in the therapeutic province of the physician. Sulfa, the treatment of choice in most instances, requires a physician's prescription. In our study, all the computer-generated prescriptions were signed by one of the doctors.

We hope this will be but a temporary expedient, however, required to conform with current regulations. I can think of no good reason why patients with uncomplicated urinary tract infection cannot prescribe for themselves, at least with the help of the computer. And the results of our study corroborate this judgment. If problems such as urinary tract infection can be managed in the home instead of the clinic, the cost savings will be substantial—and the quality of care can be at least as good, if not better. And more and more people are working to develop such programs. There is good work being done in a number of academic settings, including Case Western Reserve University, Dartmouth Medical School, Massachusetts General Hospital, the Mayo Clinic, and the University of Wisconsin. The field is becoming active.

—⁓—

I used to dream of what I called the interactive Benjamin Spock, a computer-based program in the home that would offer advice and suggestions about prevention of medical problems, as well as diagnosis and treatment when such problems arose. The program would also help patients to seek and use health care resources and make health care decisions in an enlightened manner. With such a program, patients could more easily participate as partners with clinicians in medical decisions. The computer would not replace the doctor; it would fill a void. Patients must make medical decisions for themselves all the time, sometimes the most difficult ones, such as when to go to the doctor. My hope was that the computer would be available to help people make these decisions in a more knowledgeable and enlightened manner.

Now, with more and more PCs available to more and more people, and the technology of nationwide and worldwide communication over the Internet, this dream is becoming a reality. Web sites offer a wide range of health-related information. And we are working to get our programs into the home by means of the Internet. But there are formidable barriers to overcome. Developing good interactive programs is difficult and expensive, and those of us in the field have a lot of work to do.

Before moving on to the Internet, let me turn first to studies of the computer in psychology and psychiatry—a somewhat controversial field, to say the least.

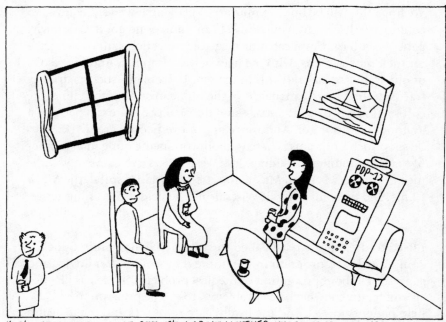

"HE'S NOT MUCH TO LOOK AT, BUT HE'S A GREAT LISTENER, UNDERSTANDS MY DEEPEST NEEDS, AND DOESN'T GOLF."

CHAPTER FOUR

Cybermedicine in Psychology and Psychiatry

⸺◟◞⸺ S ince the early 1960s, the computer has been applied with increasing frequency to the fields of psychology and psychiatry. One of the first applications, at the Mayo Clinic, was to use the computer to score the results of the Minnesota Multiphasic Personality Inventory (MMPI), the most time-honored of diagnostic personality tests. The inventory was administered manually but processed by computer, which was programmed to print descriptive phrases about the patient's personality in addition to the numerical scores for use by the psychologist. It turned out, however, that the early printouts sounded pejorative. There were no favorable comments, even for patients with no emotional problems, and when patients had the chance to read the reports, they objected. In Madison at the time, I began to develop the Wisconsin Uniphasic Personality Inventory (WUPI), which would say only positive things about a person. The WUPI was never implemented, but personality tests, including the MMPI, are much less critical of people than they used to be—all part of the patient power movement, I would contend.

A PSYCHIATRY INTERVIEW

In 1968, Maxie Maultsby and I ventured into a field that was more controversial than our other computer interviews at the time. We developed a computer-based psychiatric interview, designed as a general review of behavioral problems, and introduced it to sixty-nine volunteers who had been scheduled for psychiatric evaluation. As with other computer histories, the patients reacted favorably. They indicated a slight preference for the computer as an interviewer in comparison with doctors in their experience. Some patients responded yes to preferring the doctor *and* yes to preferring the computer, apparently not wanting to hurt the feelings of either and nicely demonstrating that human beings are not always Aristotelian in their logic. They also found the computer to be more thorough. And, once again, these patients were sometimes more comfortable with the computer than they were with the clinician while answering questions of a potentially embarrassing or emotionally painful nature.

The consensus among the nine participating psychotherapists was that routine computerized psychiatric histories, if available, would add a valuable dimension to their diagnostic evaluations.

Research with the computer as a psychiatric interviewer continued at the University of Wisconsin under the direction of John Greist, and the field became increasingly active in the decades to follow, with studies of the computer in psychiatry and psychology in institutions throughout the world as well as in our Center for Clinical Computing in Boston.

As for personality tests, it is now common to have the computer actually administer them. Nicholas Covino, John Levine, Hollis Kowaloff, our colleagues, and I have been doing this at Beth Israel Deaconess Medical Center as part of the hospital-wide CCC cybermedicine system; inventories for depression, anxiety, and problems with alcohol are all conducted by patient-computer dialogue, with a high degree of patient satisfaction.

PSYCHOTHERAPY

The most common use of the computer in the clinical setting has been to collect information directly from the patient to help the psychologist and psychiatrist with both diagnosis and treatment. But the computer has also been used for psychotherapy, more commonly as an adjunct to the human therapist, but sometimes as a therapist on its own. Most computer-based psychotherapy has been done as research, in academic medical centers rather than in clinical settings. Computer-based psychotherapy is still in its infancy, but the future is bright.

In one of the earliest ventures into psychotherapy, back in the 1960s, Joseph Weizenbaum, Kenneth Colby, and their colleagues wrote computer programs (Weizenbaum's was called Eliza after Shaw's heroine in *Pygmalion*) that took messages typed by the user, rephrased them with words of similar meaning, and responded in a manner suggestive of the nondirective psychotherapy first proposed by Carl Rogers.

Since then, a number of good programs have been developed and studied, and a wide variety of theoretical approaches have been employed. John Greist and his colleagues at the University of Wisconsin employed cognitive behavioral therapy in their program. First elucidated by Aaron Beck and his coworkers, cognitive therapy consists of three parts: the didactic component, in which the therapist explains the approach to be taken (for example in the treatment of depression); the cognitive component, in which the therapist elicits the patient's thoughts at the moment and helps the patient analyze the underlying maladaptive assumptions contributing to the depression; and the behavioral component, in which the therapist helps the patient schedule thoughts and activities to supplant the depression.

Written in Converse by Paulette Selmi, the Wisconsin program emulates the cognitive therapist. In a comparative study, the computer performed impressively—as well as the human therapist in reducing scores on tests of depression. Computer-based cognitive behavioral therapy has also been used with some reported success for patients with early Alzheimer's disease and stuttering problems.

Interactive voice response systems, with the telephone as the medium of therapeutic interaction between patient and computer, show great promise as a means of reaching a large number of people; they can be accessed from the patient's home or portable phone at any time of day or night. In a large, randomized controlled trial, Lee Baer, John Greist, Isaac Marks, and their colleagues have studied this approach using principles of behavior therapy for patients with obsessive compulsive disorders, and the results have been encouraging. They have also studied a similar program using cognitive behavioral therapy for depression with encouraging preliminary results.

There is also a growing use of the Internet for "on-line therapy," whereby patients and psychotherapists communicate with each other by means of chat groups, newsgroups, and e-mail. But this is subject matter for another book.

Virtual Environments

Sometimes called "virtual reality," virtual environments date back to World War II, when Edwin Link and Luis DeFlorez introduced the simulated airplane, which could be used for pilots in training without risk to human or machine; most airlines now use computer-based virtual cockpits for pilot training. But now, with the computer and miniature components, the equipment for the virtual environment can be worn on your head and hands as you move about, as shown on the movie screen in Michael Crichton's *Disclosure*. Picture the guy with the high-tech headset—replete with goggles, miniature TV screens (with computer-based pictures of the simulated environment), and three-dimensional sound—and proprioceptive gloves that send information about hand movements back to the computer. With a computer and the right equipment, you can navigate through multiple remote environments while staying pretty much in place.

One of the most promising applications of the virtual environment has been its use in the treatment of phobia. By simulating the offending environment, the virtual environment enables the therapist to employ behavior therapy—habituating the patient by means of simulated exposure. For example, Barbara Rothbaum and her colleagues at Emory University in Atlanta have effectively treated acrophobia by gradually exposing patients to greater and greater virtual heights in the safety of the lab. They have also had encouraging results using "virtual reality exposure" for other phobias, such as fear of flying, and they are exploring this approach for the treatment of a variety of anxiety disorders.

Let me turn now to my own experience with the computer in psychotherapy, with a brief preamble about emotionally laden topics.

EMOTIONALLY LADEN TOPICS AND THE COMPUTER

In traditional psychotherapy, topics of major psychological importance are thought to be often the most unpleasant and hence the most difficult to discuss. For psychotherapy to be effective, the reluctance to unearth or discuss such difficult topics must be removed. This tenet is held whether the reluctance is interpreted as resistance to abreaction—bringing emotionally laden topics from the unconscious to open discussion (in accordance with the psychoanalytic concepts of Freud)—or the weakening of a conditioned response in the absence of reinforcing stimuli (in accordance with the behaviorist concepts of John Watson and B. F. Skinner). Furthermore, it is generally assumed that this resistance must be removed by means of the relationship established between patient and therapist.

Under some circumstances, however, resistance to such communication is diminished when it occurs in the absence of the human clinician, including the psychotherapist. This has been our experience. Even when patients are eager for their doctor to be informed, direct communication about emotionally charged issues is sometimes difficult, and indirect communication by means of the computer can be easier.

This phenomenon, which I would call abreaction with the computer, has been corroborated by others: in one study, patients undergoing treatment for alcoholism found it easier to report high levels of alcohol consumption to the computer than to a psychiatrist; in another, volunteers were more likely to reveal sexual problems to the computer than to a psychiatrist; and in a third, patients were more likely to communicate to the computer about a past criminal record, impotence, attempted suicide, and being fired from a job. And Steven Locke, our coworkers, and I have demonstrated that a computer-based screening interview could elicit more HIV-related factors in the health histories of potential blood donors than the standard questionnaire and interviewing methods currently in use at the Red Cross.

In each of those studies, however, the keyboard was the means of communication. What about talking aloud?

TALKING THERAPY

In 1971, I teamed up with my brother, Charles, who is a psychologist. We wanted people to be able to talk during a computer interview. Charles and I had the idea that the computer could facilitate talking therapy, that it could encourage people to talk out loud about matters of importance to them.

Talking Aloud Alone

Back in the late 1950s, in the Psychology Department at Harvard during that wild psychedelic era of Timothy Leary and friends, Charles had experimented with soliloquy. He had equipped a tape recorder with a device that emitted a repetitive click in response to sustained sound. It also tallied the number of clicks. Charles then employed teenaged gang members from Cambridge to help him with his study. As long as the subjects in the experiment talked into the microphone, they could hear and see the counter adding up points at a steady rate, but whenever they stopped talking for more than a normal pause, the counter also ceased to give points. At the end of each experimental session of talk, each subject was paid according to the number of points accumulated during the session. The system worked well to initiate and maintain talk without a human listener in the room. Portions of the resulting tape recordings were indistinguishable from those of interpersonal interviews, and some of the participants said they felt better for having talked this way.

In the meantime, James Webb at Ohio University showed that people would talk alone when encouraged to do so by a standardized series of prerecorded (auditory) nondirective statements presented in a fixed sequence whenever there was a pause in the subject's speech. Expanding on this technique, Michael Dinoff and his colleagues at the University of Alabama promoted talk on the part of experimental subjects (including hospitalized patients) in response to fifteen requests from a prerecorded, videotaped interviewer who appeared on a screen whenever the person paused for two seconds. With this "talking alone" research, however, the stimuli promoting talk were presented in a predetermined sequence without branching; no use was made during the interviews of information provided by the person. In most clinical situations, by contrast, information obtained from the patient is used in subsequent conversation.

Speech-Understanding Systems

Computer-based speech-understanding systems are complex, expensive, limited in capabilities, and not yet readily available except in rudimentary form. Some systems can "comprehend" single words and short phrases, but sustained, protracted speech remains a difficult challenge.

Charles and I had the idea that the computer did not *have to* understand what was being said to help people help themselves. In other words, the computer could facilitate beneficial soliloquy.

The Talking Cure

Talking therapy, or the "talking cure," as Anna O. first called it in 1881, has a respected place in Western medicine. Ever since the first century A.D., when the Roman physician Celsus recommended the doctor-patient relationship as a treatment for depression and mania, dialogue between doctor and patient has had a major role in psychotherapy. Although there are important theoretical and practical differences between the various schools of talking therapy, all hold to the premise that the presence of the therapist and the relationship that results are essential to the therapeutic process.

There are problems with talking therapy as traditionally practiced, however. Typically, many sessions are required for treatment; few patients can afford the cost, and third-party payers—particularly those in the business of managed care—are reluctant to finance long-term therapy. Furthermore, hard-to-control variables, so important to the art of human discourse, lend uncertainty to scientific study and to our knowledge of how or whether desired goals are achieved through clinical conversation. Standards of comparison for controlled studies are difficult to establish. Therapists, even within the same school of thought, differ from each other and are themselves inconsistent. And the interested therapist, motivated to corroborate clinical judgment and theoretical doctrine, may bring bias to the session and unwittingly communicate it by verbal and nonverbal cues, and thus evoke responses that conform to expectations.

COMPUTER-ASSISTED SOLILOQUY

The computer is more easily subjected to the rigors of scientific investigation than the traditional dialogue between therapist and patient. Charles and I had three hypotheses. First, that the presence of a therapist is not essential in talking therapy, because patients will talk aloud alone about matters of psychological importance; second, that speaking out, as opposed to thinking quietly, is important to the effectiveness of psychotherapy; and third, that the doctor-patient relationship, although often beneficial, can sometimes inhibit frank disclosure. In the latter case, soliloquy can be more effective than dialogue with a therapist.

We reasoned that text on a computer screen could be a good stimulus for talk and that keyboard responses could be used to select text that would encourage talk about subjects of relevance to the person. Accordingly, we developed a computer program capable of controlling a tape recorder (and sensing when someone was talking into it) in conjunction with conducting a medical interview. With this program, people could be encouraged to talk about their own problems, and recorded messages could be left for the doctor.

We used a PDP-12 computer (Digital Equipment's successor to the LINC) connected electronically to the control unit and microphone of a tape recorder—old-fashioned technology by today's standards, but it worked well for our purposes. (Robert Herman, a medical student at the time, did the computer programming for us.) The user's responses determined the questions presented next. The time elapsed after the display of a question and intervals between points of reference in the interview could also be used as conditions for proceeding or not proceeding.

The occurrence of sound (as sensed at the microphone) was relayed to the computer and was available as another contingency for presenting new text on the screen. There was *no* comprehension by the program of what was actually said. The computer could only detect the presence or absence of sound. However, information obtained by keyboard responses during the course of the interview could be used as the basis for encouraging the user to talk, and the event of talk (or lack of it) could be used to determine what would subsequently appear on the screen. The tape recorder was under computer control and could be turned on whenever speech was being encouraged. Recordings of all discussion with the computer were thus available to us for transcription and analysis.

The Interview

The interview, which was initially designed for men, opened with words of welcome and instructions telling how to interact with the computer. These were followed by a series of medical-history questions dealing with common emotional problems beginning with sadness. ("Have you been feeling sad or down in the dumps?") If the answer was yes, the respondent was told that he would have an opportunity to discuss this sadness later on if he wished. The program then asked about the loss of someone close, loneliness, social or marital problems, problems with parents, problems at school, difficulty with self-expression, problems of a sexual nature, problems with drugs, and insomnia.

After the medical-history questions, the computer asked if the user was willing to discuss his sadness ("You indicated that you have been feeling sad; are you willing to talk a bit about this?") or whichever of the problems, if any, was detected in the interview. If so, the tape recorder was turned on automatically, and the program presented a statement encouraging talk about the problem. If the user delayed, he was asked if he was having trouble getting started, and if so, he was given advice on how to begin. The user responded to most questions by means of the keyboard; when he spoke, he did so into the microphone located between the screen and the keyboard.

As soon as talk was sensed by the computer, the program branched to a statement that acknowledged and encouraged the discussion. If the user paused without indicating that he wanted to stop, the program asked him to tell what he thought was most responsible for the problem and later what, in his opinion, would be most helpful. Next, the computer presented statements that encouraged discussion about personal feelings at the moment; something about the respondent that could not possibly be true; a personal problem considered in a very rational way; and an example of behavior that, in the respondent's opinion, was a "responsible act"—topics considered important to the psychology of Carl Rogers, Freud, Albert Ellis and Maxie Maultsby, and William Glasser. Discussion was acknowledged with words such as "We are 'listening' to you talk about. . . . If finished, press 'GO.'" Once again, delays in getting started and prolonged pauses during discussion resulted in explanation and encouragement. A person could refuse to discuss anything suggested by the computer and could leave a topic at any time.

An Experimental Trial

Thirty-two men between the ages of eighteen and twenty-six (none of whom were currently receiving psychotherapy) were recruited through colleges and medical schools in the Boston area and paid to participate in the experiment. Each subject was interviewed by one of us, as well as by the computer, half interacting first with the computer, and half first with one of us. We attempted to follow basically the same protocol as the one followed by the computer, and our interviews were also recorded on tape. Inadvertently, the question concerning the loss of someone close was omitted from our (human) questioning. In each setting discussion of a problem detected by history was limited to ten minutes, and discussion of each of the topics relating to the schools of psychotherapy was limited to five minutes.

The volunteers came to our laboratory three times: for an orientation session, at which the design of the experiment was explained with emphasis on the fact that the computer would not understand what was being said and recorded; for the experimental interviews; and for an evaluation session when each subject was asked, by written questionnaire, a series of questions regarding his reaction to the interviews. Each subject then met with us for an informal consideration of the experiment. All the participants gave express permission to use their recordings for analysis, demonstration, and publication, with the understanding that we would protect their confidentiality. Analysis of the content of what was said was performed by three independent observers using the "Experiencing Dimension" developed by Eugene Gendlin.

Responses to the Interviews

All thirty-two participants had something to say to the computer as well as to the doctor, and many talked in poignant ways about aspects of their lives. Life had not been easy for most of them. In talking to the computer, one subject discussed a problem with a girlfriend as follows:

> My girlfriend is emotionally unstable. She has problems with herself. She doesn't seem to be able to figure out why she's so frustrated. She has anxiety attacks. For that reason, she gets cold, frustrated, and angry over things that most people wouldn't normally get angry and frustrated about. Sometimes I think the way she feels is rubbing off on me. Sometimes I'm afraid to get too close to her for fear of my own sanity if I ever left her, or for fear of her own sanity if I ever left her. Sometimes I think I would like to wind the whole situation down and bring it to a halt. I don't know whether I stay in it because of myself or because of her. There is more, but I wouldn't want to stall any longer. [Here there was a prolonged pause followed by encouragement from the computer to discuss possible causes of the problem.] Her anxiety attacks . . . and being unable to be sure whether I can handle them or not. She goes to see a social worker, and she tells everything to the

social worker, and I think she almost feels that she can't tell the problems to me because she has this thing with the social worker being her dominant person—someone she can look up to and trust—whereas she feels she might be in some sort of competitive relationship with me, and she doesn't want to lose me. Therefore sometimes—oh, a lot of times—she's afraid to even talk to me. We have a communication breakdown and it's very frustrating. . . . I just feel that it's a great emotional strain on me . . . whereas I'm working five hours for four nights and going to school full time . . . I love the girl but I don't know whether I can handle it. [In this instance, the computer interview preceded the doctor interview.]

Emotional problems were common among the volunteers; only three of the thirty-two answered no to all the medical history questions. Of the twenty-nine people who had one or more problems as elicited by the computer or by one of the doctors, twenty-two discussed a problem with both the computer and the doctor. Twelve of these talked about their feelings of sadness, and ten discussed other problems.

Five of the participants discussed a problem only with the doctor. With two of these people, questions that had been answered negatively to the computer were answered positively to the doctor and the problems were discussed only with him. A third person did not care to talk with the computer about a sexual problem that he had already discussed with the doctor. The other two, each of whom had first established good rapport with a doctor, expressed hostility to the computer while talking to it. Later, they told us they could have communicated better with the machine if they had not seen the doctor first. The following are two excerpts from one of these discussions with the computer:

Personal feelings right now are . . . I certainly do have something that might be interesting to talk to a doctor about. It just seems very impersonal to be speaking to a machine that really shows—doesn't show any emotion or . . . I don't have anything to say to this monster here!

I suppose I could do something for somebody else in the future by maybe saying something about this computer. It just doesn't seem to relax you enough or make you feel warm enough. . . . If there is anything personal or something that is bothering you, it's hard for a person like myself to speak to a machine that's flashing green and black . . . sorry!

Two other people, whose single problem was the loss of someone close—the problem inadvertently neglected by the doctors—discussed it only with the computer.

The topics from the four schools of psychotherapy proved to be good promoters of talk for the computer, as well as for the doctors. In response to the request by the computer to discuss a personal problem in a very rational way (in accordance with the school of Ellis and Maultsby), one person said the following:

> Well . . . I'm having trouble finding out who I am . . . but I also have to take in all sides of the thing. I have to figure out what it is that makes me up . . . what differences I have from other people . . . what ways I can do things better, or not as good. I have to take into account my intellect . . . my personality . . . how I do things . . . how it affects other people . . . how I actually relate to other people. I look at it all, and you have to sit back and look at it rather objectively. You have to so detach yourself from it to see who you are and how you are relating to these other people. Ah . . . I think I do take the time to sort of look at things objectively. I can sort of remove myself actually from the . . . situation and look at it as if I were looking at another character . . . or at least I think I can.

Eight people indicated by the questionnaire and subsequent discussion that they felt more at ease while talking to the computer than while talking to the doctor. One person, when asked by the computer to discuss his personal feelings at the moment (in accordance with the nondirective approach advocated by Carl Rogers), said the following:

> Ah . . . at present I feel sort of strange. This is the first time I've ever talked to a computer or used a computer . . . Um . . . I . . . well, as far as how I understand the experiment, the primary objectives of this experiment are . . . I'll tell you my feelings talking into a computer. From what I understand . . . the experiment is to compare one's response to a series of questions asked by a computer and a series of questions asked by a doctor. At the moment I feel like I'm talking into a tape recorder. I'm not really nervous. . . . I have no qualms about talking into the recorder or into the computer. I . . . well, at the time I . . . it's something useful . . . I feel these things are going to be observed by humans, by doctors, so I feel no qualms about talking into this. In a

way I think I rather like talking to a computer. There's nobody to bother me. . . . I can say whatever I feel like and there's nobody look-ing to respond to what I say. It's sort of an indifference that is . . . that is here, and it has no effect on the way I talk as far as if you say some-thing and somebody responds in a negative manner, you tend to shy away from continuing in that line. Well, there is none of that in talk-ing to a computer . . . so I feel OK in talking to him [sic].

Variability of the Interviewer

One problem fundamental to research on the psychology of inter-viewing is the variability of the human interviewer. The same doctor may react differently to different people or at different times of the day and, by varying the interviewing technique, alter the way in which people respond to the questions. With the computer, the interviewing stimuli are consistent from person to person, and variations between people are more likely to be due to their actual differences than to the interviewing technique of the computer.

Likewise, in a study that compares people's responses over time, if the individuals are consistent in their responses to the computer inter-viewer and more varied in their responses to the doctors, this would indicate that the variability was due to changes developing in the doc-tors' technique rather than to changes in the people being interviewed. In this study, the participants were more revealing if they spoke to the doctors in the morning rather than in the afternoon, whereas they were equally revealing to the computer in the morning and afternoon. The absence of diurnal variability in computer sessions supports the interpretation that the doctors, rather than the subjects, were respon-sible for this difference and were perhaps poorer interviewers in the afternoon.

Furthermore, in the morning, when revelation in speech with the doctors was more substantive overall, it was more substantive still if the doctor interview came before the computer interview. In the after-noon sessions, however, there was more substantive revelation to the doctors among those whose computer sessions came first.

Even in a traditional clinical setting, therefore, patient-computer dialogue could facilitate subsequent dialogue with a therapist, partic-ularly if the therapist is in a relatively uncommunicative phase of the personal daily cycle.

Reactions to the Experiment

As judged by responses on the written questionnaire, the participants had varied reactions to the experiment and differed widely in their comparisons of the methods of interviewing. In general, reactions were more favorable to the human interviewers than to the computer. As designers of the experiment, Charles and I were naturally eager to have the computer do well as an interviewer. But the bias was at least in part balanced by our perceptions of ourselves as good interviewers—and perhaps even by a bit of sibling rivalry.

The attitudes of participants regarding the two interviewing situations were influenced by differences between doctors and by time of day and sequence of sessions. In general, Dr. A elicited more favorable reactions from participants in his afternoon sessions, Dr. B from those in his morning sessions. Overall, the participants seemed to relate somewhat better to Dr. A (we are not telling who is who).

Criticisms from the volunteers were helpful as we planned revisions in the program. Twenty of the thirty-two felt pressed for time while talking to the computer, and twelve indicated that they would have liked more time to talk to the machine. Accordingly, we adjusted the timing in subsequent programs in an effort to eliminate unnecessary interruptions and to put more patience into the system.

Some Thoughts About This Study

The computer in this experiment, though noncomprehending as a listener, was informed as an interviewer. It used information acquired by history questions to promote conversation appropriate to the person being interviewed. When programmed to ask specific questions about what the person has just been saying, the computer could gain information about the content and use this in prompting subsequent discussion.

The study demonstrated that people will talk to a computer about problems of importance to them and about subjects of importance to psychologists and psychiatrists, and will sometimes do so in the same way they talk to a doctor. Four of the participants thought they might have been helped by talking to the computer, and eight believed that the solitude in which they talked to the computer actually helped them verbalize their thoughts. Those who saw the computer first seemed to have an easier time talking to it than those who saw a doctor first. Perhaps the process of being referred from man to machine evoked feelings of rejection. The study did not directly address the issue of therapeutic effectiveness, however.

COMPUTER-ASSISTED SOLILOQUY IN A STUDY OF ANXIETY

In a more recent experiment designed to study the effectiveness of soliloquy with a specific emotional problem, Douglas Porter, Peter Balkin, Hollis Kowaloff, Charles, and I programmed a computer to conduct an automated interview that would address the symptoms of anxiety. In doing so, we did our best to improve the interview on the basis of our experience with earlier programs.

Once again the computer communicated in text on the screen, and the user responded at the keyboard and via a microphone beneath the screen. Again, the computer was oblivious to the meaning of spoken words, and the user was so informed. On the other hand, the machine could respond to the occurrence of speech at the microphone, to the durations of speech and silence, to the time elapsed between various points of reference in the interview, to entries on the keyboard, and to the time the user took to respond, and it could use these factors to direct the course of the interview. In addition, wire leads connected the user to a cardiotachometer, which transmitted the user's heart rate to the computer.

The interview began with words of welcome ("Hello there! Please find the <Go> key on the keyboard and press it."), followed by instructions about use of the keyboard ("The <Go> key is on the far right of the keyboard. Press it if you can."), acknowledgment and encouragement ("Exactly! Try it again."), instructions on the use of the microphone ("When the computer detects the sound of your voice at the phone, it will respond with some acknowledgment, like 'listening.' Try saying a few words."), and a request for the user's first name and for permission to use this during the interview. As a measure of anxiety at the beginning of the interview, the introductory section concluded with the Spielberger State anxiety measure, which consists of twenty questions designed to assess a person's level of anxiety at the moment.

The computer then proceeded to the section on anxiety. Introductory comments ("Most people are nervous, tense, or anxious, at least sometimes.") were followed by questions about the occurrence of anxiety when alone, with friends, with strangers, in a crowd, at a party, at school (if the user was a student), at work, and at home. Along the way, the computer encouraged the user to talk aloud about feelings ("Now tell yourself how you feel when you are anxious. Speak out loud, into the phone.") and about each of the situations in which they had occurred. Next, the computer encouraged the user to try to become anxious. ("Make a mental list of the circumstances most likely to make you anxious . . . now list them to yourself out loud.") The section concluded with a repeat presentation of the State anxiety measure.

The computer then turned to the subject of relaxation. ("You have talked about being anxious . . . now the idea is to dwell on a more comfortable state . . . relaxation.") The computer asked about the user's ability to relax under the circumstances that had been discussed in the section on anxiety, and then encouraged talking aloud about relaxation. ("Talk a bit about being at ease with strangers . . . say a little more if you can.") Then it encouraged the user to talk aloud about circumstances most conducive to relaxation and experiences with relaxation (as opposed to anxiety), and to develop and discuss strategies for relaxation in the future. The interview ended with a repeat of the State anxiety measure, a request for suggestions about the program, and thanks.

As a control for purposes of experimental comparison, we developed a "thinking interview" that encouraged the user to think quietly, as indicated by pressing a button instead of talking aloud. Otherwise, the wording and manner of presentation were identical in the two interviews. A control interview of this quality—identical in all respects except the variable being studied—is rare in studies of interviewing and was a principal strength of this experiment.

Experimental Trial

Forty-two men between the ages of twenty and thirty (none of whom were currently receiving psychotherapy) were recruited through colleges and graduate schools in the Boston area and paid to participate in the study. During preliminary sessions, the volunteers were divided into two matched groups—the talking group and the thinking group—on the basis of comparable scores on the computer-administered State anxiety and Taylor Manifest Anxiety measures and on the basis of comparable past experience with computers. At the end of the session, each volunteer was asked, by written questionnaire, about his reaction to the interviews.

Results

The two measures of anxiety improved in the experimental group but not in the control group. Both the mean heart rate and the State anxiety scores of the twenty-one volunteers in the talking group went down significantly between the beginning and the end of the interview. In the thinking group, by contrast, the drop in scores and heart rate was not statistically significant. Furthermore, the talking group spent more time talking aloud than the thinking group spent thinking quietly. During the relaxation section of the talking interview, the time devoted to talking was found to correlate significantly with both the drop in anxiety scores and the drop in heart rate—the more time spent talking, the greater the change. During the relaxation section of the thinking interview, by contrast, there was no significant correlation between the time devoted to thinking and changes in anxiety scores and heart rate. As judged by responses on the written questionnaire, the participants reacted favorably to the experiment in general, being equally well disposed to both the talking and the thinking interviews.

Implications

The primary approach with the soliloquy interview—to encourage each subject to speak first about anxiety, then about relaxation, and finally about personally developed strategies for replacing anxiety with relaxation—appears to have been effective under the experimental circumstances of this study. Encouragement to talk about relaxation was more effective than encouragement to think about it, as judged by the time devoted to each and the reductions in heart rate and State anxiety scores in the talking group. The correlations between these reductions and the time devoted to talking aloud indicate that computer-assisted soliloquy was more beneficial than thinking quietly in promoting relaxation. It would seem that talking aloud helps to keep us on track—on mental course, so to speak—when we are developing strategies that could promote our mental health.

The participants in this study were not patients; they were paid volunteers whose mean State anxiety scores at the start of the study were substantially lower than they would have been among men with the clinical diagnosis of anxiety. It is possible that computer-assisted soliloquy would have produced more striking results among patients with the symptoms of anxiety.

With the computer in our research, the variability and bias of the human interviewer can be eliminated as independent variables, and standards for comparison, such as the thinking interview for comparison with the soliloquy interview, can be more readily established. In the future, we plan to use the computer to study soliloquy further, both as an independent approach to therapy and as an adjunct to more traditional methods.

Paying our volunteers (a reversal of the usual arrangement between psychotherapist and client) did not seem to impede discussion. In fact, our subjects behaved very much like patients when discussing their problems. Still, people who come for help may react differently to the computer. The effectiveness of any of the existing approaches to talking therapy is uncertain, and it is not easy to evaluate the computer. But in spite of uncertainty about what works and what does not, psychotherapists are in demand and are often unavailable; where they are available, they are expensive. If the computer can help, and we believe it can, many people stand to benefit.

Abreaction with Computer-Assisted Soliloquy

In our first study of computer-assisted soliloquy, eight of the thirty-two volunteers indicated that "it might be easier to confess some things to the computer than to the doctor," whereas nineteen indicated "it might be easier to confess some things to the doctor." In the experiment with the anxiety program, twenty-four of the forty-two volunteers indicated that it "might be easier to talk to a computer about some things," whereas eighteen indicated it "might be easier to talk to a doctor." These responses indicate that under some circumstances (just as when they communicate with the computer by means of a keyboard), people are less resistant to *talking* about emotionally laden problems in the absence of a therapist.

SOLILOQUY IN EVERYDAY LIFE

In informal surveys, most of the people we ask indicate that they talk aloud alone, at least on some occasions. Charles and I believe that talking alone is practiced sporadically by almost everybody in our culture. On the other hand, it is practiced systematically by almost no one. Yet when we encourage people to talk aloud alone on their own, systematically when possible, they tell us they feel better for doing so.

The fact that some mental patients talk to themselves (to their benefit, in our view) does not mean that if you do, you will become a mental patient. Quite the opposite. You may find that it helps reduce emotional tensions by providing an outlet, for example, for hostility. Contrary to the common notion that soliloquy is a manifestation of mental illness, we believe that it is normal behavior—behavior that serves to help maintain emotional equilibrium. Because of its link with mental illness, however, soliloquy is not as yet socially acceptable; to be overheard talking alone can be cause for embarrassment. Even we don't recommend talking to yourself in front of others; *we* wouldn't think it was crazy, but *they* might. The trick is to get off where nobody can hear you, and then let loose.

Soliloquy therapy is probably the world's smallest school of psychotherapy, to date. But we hope it will grow, and that as a result of our studies with the computer, people will be more comfortable with soliloquy—theirs as well as others'. Just about anyone can try; it's noninvasive, and there are no known adverse side effects. And as Groucho Marx said in assessing "free love," at least the price is right.

ARE THEY TALKING TO SOMEONE?

Remarks made to a computer, in our experience, are not readily distinguished from those made to persons, even when emotional problems are at issue. The following selections from our experimental interviews—all from volunteers who gave permission to publish their remarks—contain no obvious references to the computer or the doctor. Can you tell which were told to him and which to it? (You'll find the answers at the end of this chapter.)

1. Well, my sadness primarily stems from the fact that I see so many things going on around in society, in the world, but the things that I find hard to accept and I guess that I'm somewhat of an idealist. I see things that should not be. You know when you stop and consider that civilization in various forms has been going on for the past ten thousand years, it seems rather disheartening to look around you and see that man really has not progressed. Technology has progressed but the wars are the same.

2. I generally try to stay away from sex ... ah ... with women because it's usually too much of a hassle after everything is said and done to be worth the while of going out and having sex with women.

I don't know how to really express it in more detail having been caught short without having thought about what I would say. I think I generally don't receive enough spiritual compensation to make up for the spiritual effort in any kind of a relationship with women. It's pretty impossible for me now to have any kind of meaningful sexual relationship with women.

3.   I could never be a good musician. I have no sense of rhythm. That bothers me.

4.   Well, at this moment I feel pretty well at ease although a little confused about the procedure here. I don't know, I'm a pretty well-adjusted person. Things don't tend to bother me unless they're very important to me and right now I'm in a fairly secure situation and I feel pretty well at ease. There isn't anything that's bothering me right now. I think the only feeling, the only word that could express my feelings right now is one of contentment at what I'm doing.

5.   I feel that I am in a stage in my life where I am coming to understand myself and part of this is to understand my sexual role and I'm changing mentally so, as I mature more I have to understand who I am going to be and I'm trying to adjust to who I am as I'm becoming who I will be. It's just a general problem actually, knowing who I am at the moment and ah, it's not altogether serious. I realize what I'm doing and ah, I have a pretty good hold on myself. It's just that it is a big problem understanding yourself and your sexuality.

6.   Well, recently I lost my grandfather who I was fairly close to. I'm really willing to answer any specific questions. I don't know exactly what to say. I've been closer to other people than that, but my grandfather is the closest person to me that had died. Um . . . I was prepared for his death in that he had been sick for an extensive period of time, so that, ah, his death was more of a blessing than anything else in that it ended his suffering and hopefully he is having his heavenly reward if there be one. Um . . . I guess that's really all I have to say about it, since there are no specific questions."

7.   Well, I suppose I'll begin with—my vocabulary isn't that good— my amount of words isn't that hot and ah, I can express myself when I'm writing and I get the point across, but when I'm talking I seem to mumble and stutter so ah, that's the problem.

8. [Pause.] Yeah, I have trouble expressing myself, all right. I can express myself when I'm writing, but I can't seem to do it when I'm talking; I have a little trouble. I have a limited vocabulary. I seem to stutter every time I begin to talk and that will be my problem of expressing myself.

In spite of good research with the computer as psychotherapist, it is still unusual for human therapists to employ computing in clinical practice. Before such programs become widespread, they should be carefully evaluated. Once again, my guidelines for good programs are as follows: they should be medically sound; they should be easy to use; they should be truly interactive; they should be of immediate and if possible long-range benefit to the patient; they should have the patient in charge; they should protect confidentiality; they should be readily available to people of all socioeconomic backgrounds; they should be fast and reliable; and they should be studied for effectiveness and safety. We will continue with our efforts in this direction.

Turn with me now to the technological revolution that is bringing computing to patients everywhere.

Answers to the who's-talking-to-whom quiz:

1. Computer
2. Doctor
3. Doctor
4. Computer
5. Computer
6. Computer
7. Doctor
8. Computer

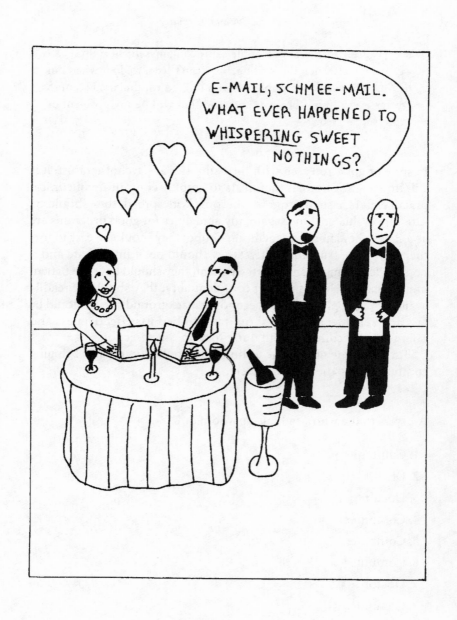

CHAPTER FIVE

The Patient On-Line

Until 1980, patients had little direct access to computing. Patient-computer dialogue was for the most part limited to research projects in academic institutions that could afford computing facilities. Computing outside of medical centers was talked about, but in futuristic parlance. As for computing in the home, this was but a dream for some and a pipe dream for others. In the 1970s, of course, television games employed computer technology, but they were toys. The original handheld calculator, the Pocketronic, was available in 1970 for $400 (more on this later)—but this was not considered a real computer by those who were enamored of the big machines. My experience with the LINC had convinced me that smaller and smaller machines would proliferate, but I didn't predict that differential equations would be computed on a handheld! Some of us took it for granted that computers would be used in the home, but as recently as the late 1970s, it was common wisdom that computers would be impractical as domestic machines.

What most people did not foresee was the personal computer, which would change our way of thinking forever. Expensive at first and with limited practical use—interactive games and spreadsheet accounting were staple fare—it caught on rapidly during the 1980s. The first major breakthrough in personal computing software was the word processor, which replaced the typewriter almost as quickly as the calculator replaced the slide rule (calculators with multiple functions were selling for $3 last time I checked). With rapidly advancing technology in its microprocessors and other inner workings, and with remarkable developments in magnetic disk storage, the PC and its derivative laptop have carried us into a vast new electronic era. The machines are getting more powerful, more portable, and less expensive as I write. It is estimated that there are well over 100 million PCs in the United States alone.

The amount of information available to us on disk has increased dramatically over the past decade, and medicine on disk has kept pace, with programs that promise sage advice and offer home remedies for a variety of ailments. Some disks are free, some are reasonably priced, and some are expensive. Some are good, some are not so good, and some are bad. It's hard to judge. I try to keep in mind my nine guidelines for judging a program, but too often there is little or no information accompanying the disk to tell us how often people use the program, how much they like it, and how well it works. Furthermore, as with printed materials, information on disks can become quickly outdated, and the user must rely on the Postal Service for new and updated versions. But I do not mean to demean this powerful technology. Programs on disks, if well written and well tested, continue to hold promise for helping people to help themselves with matters of health and disease.

It has been said, however, that the only thing constant about computing is that it changes. Consistent with this observation, there is the new technology across the land that at once has greatly expanded the number of programs available on our personal computers *and* enabled us to interact with others. This of course is the Internet.

TELECOMMUNICATION

The first computer-based telecommunication system in the United States was established in the late 1960s by the Department of Defense. The purpose was to enable workers in defense facilities to send information from facility to facility as well as to industrial centers and academic institutions involved in military projects. As the program evolved, a large network of intercommunicating computers was formed—ARPANET (Advanced Research Projects Agency Network)—that permitted nationwide electronic communication among those who were engaged in defense activities. At the heart of the network was a standardized protocol for electronic communication— TCP/IP (Transmission Control Protocol/Internet Protocol), that is still used today. TCP/IP is the agreed-upon process whereby packets of information are transmitted from one computer to another, passing en route through multiple intermediary computers and computer networks by what has been called a series of handshaking procedures.

The original purpose of ARPANET was to provide a means of sending large files of information from one computing center to another, and this proved to be a powerful form of telecommunication. Within a decade, the uses for interinstitutional communication, real and potential, had extended far beyond the ambit of any military objectives.

In the early 1980s, the NSF (National Science Foundation) replaced the Department of Defense as the principal source of government funding for this rapidly growing system. With ARPANET as the electronic framework, the NSF sponsored the development of a nationwide network, soon to be called the Internet, that would link smaller networks of computers in government departments, state as well as federal, together with industrial and academic research centers; the NSF offered grants to support colleges and universities in their effort to develop their own networks and link them to the Internet. The NSF and, later, the National Aeronautics and Space Administration (NASA), then developed "very high-speed Backbone Network Services" (vBNS) with great capacity for transmitting large amounts of information from one supercomputer to another along the Internet, thereby greatly enhancing the powers of communication. Soon, private companies began to sponsor the development of their own networks for access to the Internet, and before long, large corporations—eventually called Internet Service Providers (ISPs)—were building their own vBNS and using them to market access to the Internet by smaller organizations and individuals, who could sign on if they were equipped with personal computer, TCP communication software, modem, and telephone line.

The Internet is a remarkably egalitarian technology, functioning without centralized control and open to more and more people from all walks of life. Free of hierarchical management, the Internet is a loose federation of many thousands (probably millions) of individual networks, locally managed and for the most part self-supporting. The primary requirement for "membership" is the willingness to adhere to the TCP/IP standards for communication, which in turn are loosely managed by members of the Internet Society, volunteers from among those who develop, enhance, and maintain the communication protocols. Criticized in years gone by as a closed-minded group of computerniks, the Internet Society now eschews high-tech elitism and works toward the goal of open access. Members of the society may differ on technical issues, but they share a common commitment to democratic principles.

The World Wide Web

The File Transfer Program (FTP), one of the most powerful technical capabilities of the Internet, permits transfer of files from one computer to another at the beck and call of any user. Accordingly, millions of data repositories on a wide range of topics are available to each and every person who signs on to the Internet. The list of subjects, from aardvark to Zulu, and in medicine, from abdomen to zygote, is encyclopedic in scope. On the other hand, when you are looking for information of specific relevance to your interests at the moment, the logistics of searching can be a formidable, often bewildering, task. Raw access to the Internet is not friendly.

It is common in computing for easy-to-use programs to be needed to help with access to difficult-to-use ones, and a number of programs have been developed to ease access to the Internet. Telnet, for example, lets your computer connect to one of the computers on the Internet and behave as if it were a terminal; Gopher, developed at the University of Minnesota and named after the university mascot, offers access to resources on the Internet by a series of menus; and, with extension of the nomenclature to the entire biological order Rodentia, Veronica (very easy rodent-oriented netwide index to computerized archives) indexes the Gopher menus and allows the user to search the menus for words. Programs such as these have found widespread use in academic and industrial settings.

The newest and for almost all users now the best method for using the Internet is the World Wide Web (WWW). First developed at the European Particle Physics Laboratory in Geneva, Switzerland, the Web consists of a large and rapidly growing number of sites on the Internet that are easy to get to, easy to use, and pleasing to the eye.

Special utility programs are available to help you negotiate the Web. Browsers such as Netscape Navigator and Internet Explorer give you quick access to the multiple sites on the Web. In turn, Web sites such as Yahoo (http://www.yahoo.com), which was one of the first of its kind, have powerful programs called "search engines" that let you explore the vast resources of the Internet by typing words representing topics of interest. And the Web has do-it-yourself capabilities; with relative ease, you can create your own site on the Internet, with text and color graphics if you wish, for others to browse. Web technology has greatly augmented the use of the Internet.

On-Line Services

During the 1980s, computer-based information services in addition to the Internet appeared on-line for use by anyone with a personal computer, modem, telephone line, and funds to pay for the service. The price has varied over the years, and now typically involves a modest monthly rate in the range of $20 per month—and a willingness to tolerate the many advertisements that accompany the programs. CompuServe, the first; Prodigy, which came later; and America Online, the newest, are the three most prominent of these telephone line services, and each offers a large array of its own programs. (CompuServe was recently purchased by America Online.) As the popularity of the Internet grew, people wanted faster communication than could be provided via telephone lines. Cable modems and digital subscriber lines (DSL) now provide such access for about $40 per month. Most colleges and universities in the United States as well as numerous public and private secondary schools now offer access to the Internet for students and faculty alike, and the number of home users is ever increasing. According to a compilation of recent surveys by Nua Internet Surveys (http://www.nua.ie/surveys), over 350 million people use the Internet worldwide, and over 150 million people use the Internet in Canada and the United States.

As a cautionary note, I might point out that browsing the Internet can be addictive. There is even a self-help group for excessive users (Web site unknown).

COMMERCE ON-LINE

Before getting to medicine on-line, let me digress for a paragraph to say a few words about business ventures on the Internet. In 1995, use of the Internet as a pathway for commerce began to surge, and *dot-coms*—named for the last part of their Web addresses—appeared in great numbers. But in spite of much optimism and an abundance of venture capital early on, Internet-based companies couldn't figure out how to generate income for their services—how to compete with the services that already offer an abundance of information to the public without charge. This remains a dilemma, and since the turn of the century, dot-coms have disappeared with even greater rapidity than they appeared. Still, if the logistics of revenue generation can be worked out, and there is good reason to believe that it can—although probably not with advertisements, which have been ineffective thus far—the dot-com industry will rise again.

MEDICINE ON-LINE

By whatever means of access, more and more medical information is available by computer-based telecommunication—that is, more and more medicine is on-line. Estimates of the number of health-related Web sites directed primarily to the patient vary widely and go as high as a hundred thousand and more. But one thing is certain; there are many of them. Yahoo, for example, offers thirteen thousand sites in response to the word "health," some of which, of course pertain to the well-being of nonmedical subjects. When you as the user home in on human health, you are presented with an opening menu (including forty-seven categories as I write, and growing all the time) in alphabetical order, beginning with Alternative Medicine, Business to Business, Chats and Forums, Children's Health, Conferences, and Death and Dying, and ending with Teen Health, Traditional Medicine, Travel Health and Medicine, Weight Issues, Women's Health, and Workplace. Each of these categories, in turn, will direct you to numerous more specific Web sites as you proceed to focus on the issue of your particular interest. If you select Women's Health, right now you get a menu of twenty-eight categories, beginning with AIDS/HIV and ending with topics such as Reproductive Health and Uterine Fibroids. If you then choose AIDS/HIV, you are directed to a list of five additional Web sites, which in turn will direct you to lists of AIDS-related newsletters compiled from a variety of sources, ranging from the Food and Drug Administration to various pharmaceutical companies.

As with all health-related literature directed to the patient, the reader must be wary of the source and seek second and third opinions. Misinformation and unfounded opinion are there along with the useful and well founded; there is very little censorship on the Internet. But the information is there in abundance, and its accessibility is unparalleled in the history of civilization. Furthermore, whenever new information is added to a Web site at its source, this information is immediately available to all who sign on to use the site; no mailings of updates are needed as they are with stand-alone disks. If we as users are careful to check the sources, we can find current, timely, and useful information on a wide range of important health-related subjects.

Health-Related Web Sites of Special Note

Three reliable sources of health-related information warrant special mention. The National Library of Medicine (NLM), a division of the National Institutes of Health (NIH) under the direction of Donald Lindberg, presents pertinent information on a wide variety of medical subjects. Its Web site (http://www.nlm.nih.gov) offers (among other categories) Health Information, which points to programs such as MEDLINEplus, which in turn directs you to a list of medical topics, from Blood/Lymphatic System, Bones, Joints and Muscles, and Cancers to Substance Abuse, Symptoms and Manifestations, Wellness and Lifestyle, and Women's Health, as well as access to a medical dictionary. If you select Blood/Lymphatic System, you get a more specific list of hematological problems from which to choose, ranging from anemia to thrombocytopenia; and if you select anemia, you are presented with multiple options that enable you to choose from the many types of anemia and then to focus on the anemia of particular interest. MEDLINEplus also provides you with the credentials and locations of doctors and dentists, state by state, as well as definitions and spellings of medical terms from a comprehensive glossary and information about the appropriate use of a broad array of medications. Health Information also offers information on a variety of additional health-related subjects, such as a directory of health-related organizations and a list of research studies currently under way that are sponsored by the NLM.

Also under Health Information, you can find access by several routes to the NLM MEDLINE database of references and abstracts from forty-three hundred biomedical journals. One of the truly outstanding contributions to come from the U.S. government, MEDLINE was originally directed to clinicians and scientists. In recent years, however, its use has expanded to a much wider audience. PaperChase, with its own Web site (http://www.paperchase.com), was the first program of its kind both to enable and facilitate direct searches of the MEDLINE database by users other than professional librarians. Paper-Chase was developed by my partner Howard Bleich and his colleagues back in the late 1970s with the support of a grant from the NLM and was in use by clinicians, patients, and prospective patients alike years before the advent of Web technology.

The Centers for Disease Control and Prevention (CDC) also offers a comprehensive array of health-related information (http://www.cdc.gov). This includes information about the CDC itself (descriptions of the eleven centers, which include epidemiology, environmental health, infectious diseases, immunizations, and occupational safety), announcements of health-related events (for example, a calendar of meetings by date, together with the person to contact), data and statistics about health and disease (for example, the leading causes of death by age—problems at birth for all people under one year, and heart problems for all people over sixty-five), "Health Topics A-Z" (with write-ups about the prevention, diagnosis, and treatment of a wide range of medical problems, from anthrax to zoster), information about health and disease as provided to the news media by the CDC (for example, a story about the supply of flu vaccine for use in years 2000 and 2001, which, although comparable in amounts to earlier years, was somewhat late in arrival), information about funds from the CDC to support research (for example, support for computing systems, of particular interest to me, I must admit), and to wrap things up, information about the numerous publications and computer programs that are available from the CDC.

Third, and perhaps the most comprehensive collection of health-related information for the general public offered by the U.S. government, is Healthfinder (http://www.healthfinder.gov) from the Department of Health and Human Services, which offers links to numerous up-to-date discussions of specific medical problems as well as more general medical issues, such as Medical Errors, Choosing Quality Care, and Fraud and Complaints. The opening Web site offers six quick reference categories: Hot Topics, with thirty timely subjects ranging from adoption, AIDS, allergies, and alternative medicine, to physical activity, pregnancy, sexually transmitted diseases, and tobacco; News, with health-related news from multiple government agencies; Smart Choices, which points to sites pertaining to self-care, choice of clinicians and clinical facilities, and readily accessible sources of on-line health information, as well as discussions of malpractice and quackery; More Tools, which directs you to medical journals and medical dictionaries; Just For You, which offers medical information for people of different age, gender, ethnicity, and occupation; and About Us, which gives you the background and goals of the Healthfinder programs. And there is more. With Healthfinder you are free to type words about subjects of particular interest and the program does its best to find them for you. If your word is not accepted, an index option will provide you with a list of acceptable words. If for example, you type "d," Healthfinder returns with fifty-eight words or phrases beginning with that letter, starting with dance therapy and ending with dystonia—with depression, diabetes, and digestive diseases along the way. Each subject can then be further qualified by age, gender, ethnicity, and first language, when such specific information is available.

There are of course a number of other health-related Web sites from reliable sources. The Medical Library Association (http://www. mlahq.org) lists, in addition to Healthfinder and the programs of the NLM and CDC, on-line sources of information it regards as especially useful: the American Medical Association's site (http://www.ama-assn.org), HealthWeb (http://www.healthweb.org) from the University of Illinois in Chicago and supported by the NLM, HIV InSite (hivin-site.ucsf.edu) from the University of California at San Francisco, Health Oasis (http://www.mayohealth.org) from the Mayo Clinic, the National Women's Health Information Center site (http://www.4women.gov), which is supported by the Department of Health and Human Services, and NOAH (http://www.noah-health.org), which bills itself as New York's "on-line access to health." I have found each of these to be a valuable source of medical information. And Harvard Medical School, my home base, now has editorial responsibility for a comprehensive Web site for consumer health information (http://www.intelihealth.com). This site offers information about wellness as well as illness and features content from the school's widely read health-related books and newsletters.

There are also many disease-specific Web sites from well-recognized, reliable, and authoritative sources, such as the Juvenile Diabetes Foundation (http://www.jdf.org), which provides a broad range of useful information for parents and children dealing with Type 1, insulin dependent diabetes. Information about such important topics as daily care and the emotional demands that confront the family with a diabetic child is offered in easily accessible, readily comprehended prose, together with strategies for dealing with the many unavoidable problems as they arise.

It becomes quickly apparent to those of us who browse cybermedicine on the Internet that there is considerable redundancy of information—and this is good, I would contend; there is safety in numbers. Furthermore, the sites I've listed often point to each other, and this in turn facilitates access.

For the most part, health-related information on the Internet is unidirectional, presented in a noninteractive and didactic manner; much of what is available on Web sites for patients is also available in pamphlets and other printed documents. Yet I am confident that as we proceed into the twenty-first century, the interactive powers of the computer will come increasingly into play, and that more and more truly interactive programs will be available that address the individual needs of the people who use them. In our laboratory here in Boston, we are working to design, implement, and study such programs.

One important solution to the rising cost of medical care is enlightened self-care in the home. And for good or for bad, patient-computer dialogue is in the home to stay.

Access to the Internet

The Internet is becoming more and more available to people of all backgrounds, in homes, schools, and workplaces. Although accurate surveys of medical use of the Internet are difficult to come by, the numbers are formidable and ever increasing. The research firm Cyber Dialogue has estimated that eighteen million Americans went on-line in search of medical information during a twelve-month period between 1997 and 1998 (http://www.nua.ie/surveys). A subsequent survey by the Pew Internet & American Life Project together with Georgetown University had the number up to fifty-five million American adults (http://www.pewinternet.org), while a survey by Louis Harris & Associates for the year 1998 had the number up to sixty million Americans, 90 percent of whom reported finding the health-related information they were looking for (http://www.nua.ie/surveys). The number could be well over a hundred million as I write. And the costs keep coming down. Once only the government and large corporate institutions could afford a computer. Now most middle-income families can afford a personal computer with modem.

As things stand now, you can go on-line for a year, with no frills, for about $1,000 and some personal guidance from someone who is already there. You can even modify your television set for Internet access for less than $500 for a year, and the price is dropping. (And if you cannot as yet afford the appropriate hardware and software, your local library probably has computers you can sign up to use.)

The health-related programs provided by the government, which of course have already been paid for with our taxes, are offered without additional charge, once you have gained access to the Internet. It is my abiding hope that access to the Internet will continue to evolve in the manner of the handheld calculator, which now almost anyone can own, and that health-related information on the Internet will someday be available for all to use when the need arises. And as we strive toward this Platonic goal, I am optimistic. The computer may have started out in the hands of the elite, but it is now available to more and more people of all backgrounds; the computer is becoming democratized as well as democratizing.

But let us turn now to what is perhaps the most powerful *and* empowering function of computer-based telecommunication—conversation by computer.

Teleconverse

Much of telecommunication is one way, with messages sent for which no reply is expected. There is a form, however, that is deserving of its own name, and I call it *teleconverse.* This is long-distance conversation—the exchange of messages between people by way of the computer. E-mail is the earliest—and still most prevalent—form of teleconverse.

In the early days of ARPANET, computer-based network technology was used primarily for sending large files of information back and forth at relatively slow rates of transmission. As things speeded up, however, messages and replies to messages were sometimes included with these packets of information. With time, short messages began to supersede large documents. Driven by its users in this way, ARPANET spawned an embryonic form of teleconverse, which within a gestational period of a few years developed into e-mail.

The best place to pave a path is where the grass is worn and people are already walking, not where you think people *ought* to walk. With computer-based telecommunication, the path being used was e-mail. No one was telling people they *had* to use e-mail; they were using it because the technology was available and it was a helpful form of day-to-day conversation. And now, with the Internet much faster than it used to be, teleconverse by e-mail has become the most heavily used of the Internet capabilities. Furthermore, virtually all the on-line services, such as CompuServe, Prodigy, and America Online, offer their own versions of e-mail, as well as access to the Internet, and multiple e-mail programs are available commercially for smaller networks of computers.

E-mail on the Internet serves many people in many different ways. Let me address a few of the health-related uses by way of example.

INDIVIDUAL MAILINGS AND POSTINGS. Any person with access to the Internet, by any means, can use e-mail. Of course you must be able to type, but since you can take all the time you want, the hunt-and-peck method works just fine. You can send me a message right now if you like, at wslack@caregroup.harvard.edu, and I will do my best to respond. You could also send a message to my colleague Tom Ferguson at doctom@doctom.com. Tom is widely recognized as a pioneer in on-line health. His newsletter (http://www.fergusonreport.com)—offered as a public service free of charge—is the best source of information about this rapidly growing field. Or you could send a message to both Tom and me at the same time, or to a larger group still. More and more people are using e-mail to communicate with each other and with their doctors about health-related matters, much to their collective benefit.

Then there are the newsgroups, which serve as electronic bulletin boards. Unlike users of personal e-mail, who receive their messages unsolicited, participants in newsgroups must request access to the postings of their group, just as they would go to a bulletin board to read messages. After reading a posted message, a user can add a comment to what has been said, introduce a new topic, or initiate a call for help. There are thousands of newsgroups, with material on a staggering number of topics, many of them health-related. Self-help groups are well represented. People with a wide variety of physical, emotional, and social problems use their newsgroups to give and receive advice and support, even in times of emergency. People contemplating suicide have turned to a newsgroup for help. Some of the groups are moderated by a person who reads and edits the incoming messages before posting them for general reading. But most of them have no moderator, so that all postings are available for all to read and respond to. (The good news is that there is no censorship with the unmoderated messages; the bad news is that extraneous and sometimes inappropriate messages can clutter or even overwhelm the group.) Messages can be personalized, however; a user can send an e-mail message directly to the originator of a posted newsgroup message to be read only by that person.

THE SELF-HELP MAILING LIST. The mailing list, as it is called in Internet parlance, is somewhat different. First there is the list owner, or facilitator, who has an interest in a particular topic, a medical topic for our purposes. The facilitator announces the formation of a mailing list on this topic, and e-mail users who share this person's interest submit their e-mail addresses as a means of becoming members. Members can send messages to the list for distribution; the facilitator either forwards the messages directly to the other members, or compiles them into an e-mail newsletter, which is then sent to members at regular intervals. With many mailing lists, an automatic mail server program compiles the messages and sends them out unedited. This saves the facilitator's time and eliminates the possibility of censorship. On the other hand, the product is often more cumbersome and less substantive than a cogent newsletter prepared by a careful editor.

Hundreds of self-help support group mailing lists are already available to those who have the equipment and inclination to search for one and sign up, and the number is growing all the time. If you are interested in a health-related topic and would like to discuss it with other people, medical or nonmedical, you can probably find an appropriate group. Were they alive, Bill W. and Dr. Bob would likely be very pleased to discover that Alcoholics Anonymous is well represented, as is Al-Anon. From AIDS and Alzheimer's disease to stroke, stuttering, and yeast infections, a large array of medical conditions are represented by on-line groups. Various Web sites, such as Topica (www.topica.com) and Yahoo Groups (www.yahoogroups.com) can help you find health-related lists of particular interest.

The following quote from Samantha Scolamiero, founder of BRAINTMR, the brain tumor mailing list, exemplifies how a mailing list can enable people to communicate as peers and help one another. This quote evolved from a series of e-mail messages and personal conversations between Samantha and Tom Ferguson. It is reprinted (with a few revisions) from Tom's book, *Health On-line: How to Find Health Information, Support Groups, and Self-Help Communities in Cyberspace,* with his permission and hers:

As a brain tumor survivor, I began BRAINTMR in 1993 with the simple hope of helping people concerned with brain tumors to share information and experiences. In a short time BRAINTMR has moved far beyond that initial vision.

Of our 1,000 members, roughly three-fourths are patients and family members. We share information and advice about the best medical centers, about little-known clinical trials, nutrition, rehabilitation, alternative therapies, doctor/patient relationships, and other resources on the Internet. Patients use printouts of list messages to get their doctors to help them join the latest clinical trials.

As one subscriber explained, "The issues and problems we deal with on the list are more specific and realistic than information gathered from books, articles, and other sources." By sources sharing wisdom gained during their brain tumor ordeal, patients and families help one another to cope and to feel empowered. The list helps to ease isolation and depression and provides a coping strategy for difficult times. People who might be intimidated by face-to-face meetings can participate in a friendly, mutually supportive exchange. BRAINTMR is a welcome haven for those with no local group. And with adaptive input/output equipment, even those who are disabled can participate.

About one-fourth of our members are neurosurgeons, nurses, psychologists, epidemiologists, pathologists, social workers, and other clinicians and researchers. Our doctor members have told me that monitoring the list helps *them* understand the specific physical, emotional, and spiritual needs of their patients [italics mine]. Such insights can be difficult in the midst of a busy clinical practice.

Countless printouts from our list circulate among brain tumor specialists. One list participant, a faculty member at a major U.S. brain tumor research center, routinely forwards list messages to forty-eight colleagues. Armed with our printouts, an oncologist in a developing country convinces colleagues to try new treatment options.

List members—laypeople and professionals alike—have moved beyond the old, obsolete mindset that holds that only certain "qualified" medical professionals may create and disseminate medical information. We are showing that we are qualified through our experience. We now see that we are capable of contributions no professional can make, and that by linking our efforts in a coordinated team, we can advance the well-being of all.

By breaking down the rigid social boundaries that traditionally exist between doctors, patients, and researchers, the BRAINTMR mailing

list is pointing the way toward a new type of participatory medicine in which *all* those concerned with a given health problem can work together as colleagues to promote healing and well-being.
Samantha J. Scolamiero
Founder and facilitator, BRAINTMR mailing list
samajane@sasquatch.com

In addition, Rand Hove, a user of BRAINTMR, wrote a series of e-mail messages to Samantha, which are summarized here with his permission:

BRAINTMR is the best service I have seen, which makes the technological commodity of electronic information intensely vital, powerful, and human. BRAINTMR is illuminating some very dark and frightening places for people who are in urgent need. Here, electronic communication has its greatest value, making us more real and tangible, as opposed to having the dehumanizing effect computers are notorious for. We are the people who are changing the definition of community for the 21st century.
Rand Hove, Brain Tumor Survivor, Minnesota

Another notable mailing list, and one of the first to emphasize patient-to-patient communication, is the list for patients, clinicians, and others with a personal interest in bone marrow transplantation (BMT-Talk). Founded by Laurel Simmons, herself a bone marrow transplant patient, BMT-Talk currently has over fifteen hundred subscribers. And the Association of Cancer Online Resources (www.acor.org), which was founded by Gilles Frydman, offers access to ninety-nine mailing lists that in turn provide information and support to over fifty thousand people with a personal interest in cancer.

Formed, maintained, and driven by users, the mailing list is patient power of the first order.

SELF-HELP CHAT GROUPS. Chat groups offer people the opportunity to converse with each other electronically at the same time. Whereas e-mail has the advantage of not requiring synchronous schedules (messages can be sent or received at any time of day or night), chat groups provide a valuable means of *real-time*—synchronous—communication. For example, one Web site offers chat group access to all who would like to communicate with others about diabetes (http://www.childrenwithdiabetes.com). Described by its founder and manager, Jeff Hitchcock, as a route to "the on-line community for kids, parents, and adults with diabetes," the Web site offers information on a wide variety of subjects of relevance to diabetes as well as access to chat groups for people with a particular interest in diabetes, such as parents, kids, pre-teens, teens, siblings, and friends. It is operated and maintained by a group of twenty-three full-time volunteer health care professionals together with thirteen part-time experts in diabetes who are available to answer questions posed by users and to make sure of the quality of the clinical information on the site.

Drawing on their personal experience, members in a chat group discuss general issues and specific problems; they ask and answer questions, and they offer and receive advice and suggestions, all in a gentle, informal, nondirective yet supportive manner, consistent from my perspective with the principles espoused by Carl Rogers. As the grandfather of a six-year-old who has had diabetes since he was seventeen months old (more about this in the epilogue), I have entered the "parents' room" and have found the dialogue with the others to offer me new insight into the day-to-day care of children with diabetes as well as demonstrating to me the power of this new medium of teleconverse. I usually find five to ten members conversing informatively with each other at any one time, and doing so with enthusiasm, verve, and wit. A mother with two diabetic teenagers wrote, "Warner, this is a SUPER place, a model of what a medical site should be"; a second mother chimed in, "Warner, this has been a huge help already to me, even though I only discovered the site a few days ago," and a third mother, in reference to a member who had been providing her with continuing support via the chat group, wrote that she "is great . . . She has helped ease me through some scary nights . . . thanks again." As Jeff Hitchcock points out so well, "Simply knowing that you're not alone can make a big difference."

Good News and Bad

As with all forms of communication, there are bad messages on e-mail as well as good ones. People have a natural tendency to single out the problems with new technology as if they were unique, when upon reflection it is clear they were part of the old technology as well. People worry about rudeness on the Internet, and it is there. But so is there rudeness on the telephone. Good manners do not always prevail with e-mail, but this is not the fault of the *medium;* it is the fault of the *message.* We should insist on courtesy as we interact with others on e-mail.

Not all mailing lists work out as a member might hope. There may be too many messages to read; messages may be useless, angry (*flaming,* in Internet parlance), or insulting. On the other hand, unsubscribing is as easy as subscribing. Membership is voluntary. And if you don't like what you see, you can always start your own mailing list. Furthermore, when Web sites are supervised, managers or governing bodies can bar access to users deemed offensive. Teleconverse on the Internet is the First Amendment in action; it is participatory democracy at its best.

No government regulatory agency exists for mailing lists as yet, and I hope there never will be. In the spirit of self-help, let us let the Internet remain self-regulatory.

E-mail is a powerful means of communication. It is impossible to estimate with accuracy the number of medically related messages that flow between people, day in and day out, but it is clearly enormous.

Early prophets of doom—"patients will refuse to have anything to do with a computer"—have been proved wrong. The burgeoning use of the Internet for medical matters attests to the fact that patients *like* to be on-line. And if they don't, they don't have to be. But what about the clinician?

Cybermedicine and the Clinician

EVOLUTION OF AN ALARMIST

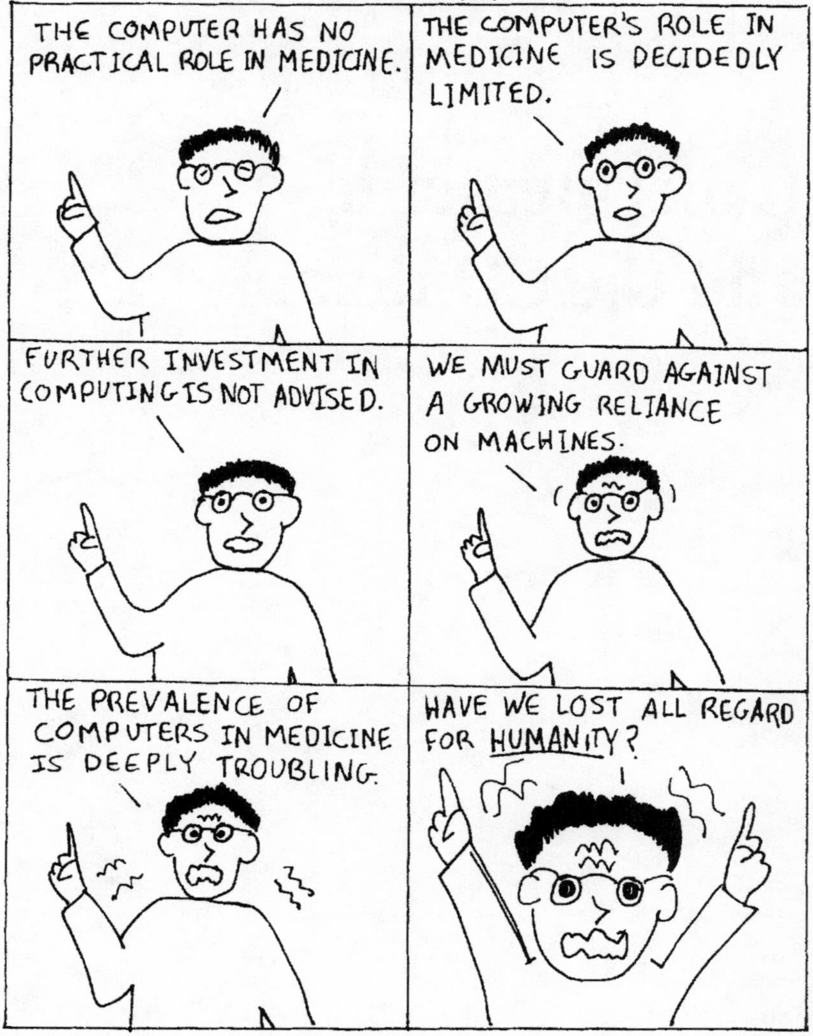

Cybermedicine in the Hospital and Clinic

I n spite of a tendency to be conservative, twentieth-century physicians tended to be liberal in their use of new technology. Unfortunately, as we learned along the way, technological innovations in medicine sometimes do more harm than good. As I have noted earlier, X rays were used to treat enlarged thymus glands, ringworm, and acne before the dangers of irradiation were well known. I can remember the fluoroscope machines that were put in shoe stores so that customers could watch the bones of their feet moving inside their shoes. Repeated exposure to the X rays could make a person—particularly a child—more susceptible to cancer. (Fortunately, the machines didn't last long in the stores, and, of course, we weren't buying shoes every day.) We must proceed with caution as we use any new technique, including the computer, in the care of patients.

On the other hand, sometimes the most notable side effect of a technological innovation is the break with tradition that its use entails. This is not likely to be of concern to the individual patient, who is interested primarily in getting well, or the individual doctor, who is interested primarily in helping patients get well, but from a collective standpoint, altering the status quo can be disturbing. After René Laënnec invented the stethoscope in 1816, physicians stopped placing an ear against the patient's chest, ending a long tradition. The change was criticized in the London *Times:* "That [the stethoscope] will ever come into general use notwithstanding its value is extremely doubtful, because its beneficial application requires much time and gives a good bit of trouble to the patient and to the practitioner, and because its hue and character are foreign and opposed to our habits and associations. There is something even ludicrous in the picture of a grave physician proudly listening through a long tube applied to the patient's thorax."

Just as the now-anonymous voice in the London *Times* worried about the use of the stethoscope in medicine in the nineteenth century, others worry about the use of the computer in medicine. In the early 1960s, with the increased availability of digital computers, many doctors were concerned about the potential encroachment of this new technology on the profession of medicine and on the traditional rapport between doctor and patient. Well-meaning Luddites among us were ready to suppress any electronic addition to the practice of medicine. The debate was frequently lively, and a commonly asked question was, "Will your computer replace the doctor?" My favorite rejoinder (borrowed from psychologists working with teaching machines) was that any doctor who could be replaced by a computer deserved to be.

IS THE COMPUTER IMMORAL?

Some among us today still worry about the computer in medicine, particularly if to use the computer is to alter the doctor-patient relationship. To them the doctor-patient relationship has intrinsic value, independent of diagnosis and treatment, and any program that interferes with this relationship should be avoided, regardless of its potential benefit to the patient.

Consider for a moment the program Eliza, which (as I have mentioned earlier) took messages typed by the user, rephrased them with words of similar meaning, and responded in a manner suggestive of the nondirective psychotherapy first proposed by Carl Rogers. Developed by Joseph Weizenbaum of MIT in the 1960s, the program was impressive for its time, and those who tried it found it interesting and entertaining. Later, however, in the tradition of Mary Shelley's fictional creator, Weizenbaum stepped back from his console and attributed dangerousness to his program. After that, he argued against the use of interactive programs in medicine, including some of mine.

Focusing on a system (similar to his own) developed by Kenneth Colby and colleagues, Weizenbaum expressed particular concern about the use of computers for psychotherapy, which he considered not only dangerous but immoral—indeed, "simply obscene." He wrote, "These are [programs] whose very contemplation ought to give rise to feelings of disgust in every civilized person. I would put all projects that propose to substitute a computer system for a human function that involves interpersonal respect, understanding, and love in this category. I therefore reject Colby's proposal that computers be installed as psychotherapists, not on the grounds *that such a project might be technically infeasible* [italics mine], but on the grounds that it is immoral."

Most of the patients I have known, "civilized" or not, would value relief from illness more highly than a relationship with a therapist. Yet Weizenbaum appears to think that the possibility of obtaining respect, understanding, and love in the clinic is more important. Does he really mean to say that if an interactive computer could help a patient with anxiety or depression (or cancer or AIDS) that would be obscene?

If therapy based on an interpersonal relationship is the best we have to offer, and certainly for some medical problems this is the case, then respect and understanding (perhaps sometimes even love) are essential to the relationship. Of course, respect and understanding are important in *all* interactions between doctor and patient, even when procedures such as patient-computer dialogue are to be used in conjunction with the clinician's care. But if an approach to therapy, with or without the computer, can be shown to be more effective, less costly, or more convenient than therapy based on a doctor-patient relationship, I think most patients would take their chances on finding respect, understanding, and love outside the clinic.

The problem is not, as Weizenbaum and those who share his philosophy erroneously conclude, that computers in medicine are dangerous or immoral; the problem is that they have yet to reach their full potential. Instead of attacking the *idea* of using patient-computer dialogue in clinical care, which even Weizenbaum knew might be technically feasible, let those of us in the field concentrate our efforts on developing programs that work well on behalf of the patient.

A HISTORICAL PERSPECTIVE
OF CYBERMEDICINE

Coupled with early concerns about the computer in medicine was excessive admiration. There is a sociological principle, often true, that people tend to react to new technology with unreasonable expectations as well as fear. The electronic digital computer, with its capacity to hold and process large amounts of information with great speed and accuracy, was indeed an awe-inspiring device—one that stimulated comparisons with the brain itself and fostered remarkable prophecies.

For most people, fear of the computer in medicine waned as the great expectations increased and prophecy became a substitute for accomplishment. Computer manufacturers, in turn, moved to capitalize on these great expectations. Some advertised their machines as panaceas for the medical community; they sold what they called total hospital information systems that were at best partial and contained remarkably little information. When the dust settled, in part on expensive, unused computer terminals, hospitals that had purchased these systems found that they had spent a great deal of money and received little in return—usually partially working billing systems. From the patient's perspective, the principal difference was that the bills, although higher because of the computing costs, arrived, if at all, somewhat *later* than before.

Typically, financial data were recorded throughout the hospital on pieces of paper, aggregated in a data processing area, keypunched onto Hollerith cards or magnetic media, and fed to the computer. From these data, the computer produced bills for patients or third-party payers, payment checks for the hospital's creditors and employees, and a very large number of printed reports. Computers programmed to handle batches of financial transactions have proved poorly suited to interactive clinical applications, and have had little impact on the practice of medicine.

Pioneers in Cybermedicine

In the 1960s, however, a small but growing number of people from the United States, Canada, Great Britain, Europe, and Asia, primarily clinicians and computer scientists in medical schools and teaching hospitals, began to work actively with computers in medicine. Virtually all clinical computing in those days was restricted to large machines in large clinical institutions. There were no desktop—let alone laptop—computers.

Supported for the most part by government grants, these pioneers got their own machines and used principles from a wide variety of disciplines, including arithmetic, symbolic logic, Boolean logic, algebra, probability, linguistics, statistics, and the theory of games. They studied the computer as a diagnostician; as an interpreter of images such as electrocardiograms, electroencephalograms, and X-ray films; and as a teaching machine for students and clinicians in training. And they demonstrated that the needs of individual clinical departments such as the admitting office, the medical records department, the pharmacy, the pathology department, and the radiology department could successfully be served by computers. With few exceptions, these programs were electronically isolated from one another, or interfaced in such a manner that they could not readily share information, yet they pioneered the introduction of computing into the hospital environment.

Also in the 1960s, stand-alone computers began to appear in the laboratories of hospitals and clinics. They were used to collect test results from automatic analyzers, print results on paper forms for distribution to clinicians for use in patient care, assist in maintaining the accuracy of diagnostic machines that produced the results (a process called quality control), and capture charges for use in billing patients or their third-party payers. To this day, many hospitals and clinics have such computing systems in one or more of their laboratories and clinical departments.

The Chip in the Laboratory

The evolution of the automatic analyzers in the clinical laboratories, the diagnostic machines used in clinical departments such as cardiology, neurology, and radiology, and the diagnostic machines now available for patients to use in their homes (the glucometer, for example, but more of this later) is a story of rapidly advancing computer technology of a different nature. Embedded in these machines are the chip and microchip, the building blocks of all computers, containing large amounts of electronic circuitry. The machines used for diagnostic *procedures,* such as electrocardiography (ECG) and cardiac catheterization in the cardiology department; electroencephalography (EEG) and electromyography (EMG) in neurology; and X rays, ultrasound, magnetic resonance imaging (MRI), and, by definition, computerized axial tomography (CAT scanning) in radiology, all have built-in computers.

The CAT scan and MRI, which provide exquisitely detailed images of soft tissues, organs, and organ systems, are high on my list of important medical inventions of the twentieth century. These noninvasive methods have replaced draconian procedures such as the pneumoencephalogram. Used to detect lesions, such as tumors, in the brain, the pneumoencephalogram involved withdrawing spinal fluid with a needle and replacing it with air. The air would then fill the ventricles of the brain, permitting the structures to be seen on X-ray. Having done this painful, lengthy, and potentially dangerous procedure on children as well as adults, I particularly appreciate the new machines.

On a related subject, the practice of medicine entails numerous calculations—often laborious and sometimes error-laden—and for the most part clinicians have been quick to adopt any machine that would help with numeric processes.

The Handheld Computer

The pursuit of extracerebral assistance in manipulating numbers is not new. Fingers (or toes) were probably the first adding machines. These in turn most likely gave rise to our decimal orientation, including our tendency to prescribe medications in regimens of ten days, regardless of their pharmacology.

Irene Kim has written an informative review of the evolution of inanimate calculators, from the abacus—the first handheld calculator invented some twenty-five hundred years ago—to the miniature handheld of today. During the first half of the twentieth century, calculators were still Pascal-type machines, mechanical in design, even when they were electrically powered. Those of us who went to college before the 1970s remember all too well the Monroe desktop calculator with the four arithmetic functions, powerful for its time but scarce in supply—typically, one or two to a college department—along with a sign-up sheet and a long waiting time.

The invention of the transistor by John Bardeen, W. H. Brattain, and William Shockley in 1948 led to the development of the first truly electronic (all-transistor) calculator in 1964. Manufactured by Sharp

Electronics, this machine, which performed the arithmetic functions, weighed fifty-five pounds and sold for $2,500. (The slide rule was still much in evidence.) I remember at the time predicting that someday the price and size of such machines would come down—that you would be able to afford your own calculator and take it home in your briefcase. I did not predict that you would be able to get one that would fit in your wallet—for $1 and a Wheaties box top.

In 1958, Jack Kilby of Texas Instruments invented the integrated circuit. Seven years later, he began to think seriously of a truly portable electronic calculator, one small enough to hold in your hand—too small to be made with transistors but perhaps it could be made with integrated circuits. And together with his colleagues at Texas Instruments, he set out to build one.

Kilby was confronted with formidable problems as he embarked on the project. There were difficulties with the circuitry (the quality of the chips was inconsistent and it was difficult to make reliable contacts between the necessarily large number of leads), with the power supply (he insisted on a battery for portability, and a heavy silver-zinc battery was the best available), and with the display (a small thermal printer was eventually used). But in 1967, prototype literally in hand, Kilby and his colleagues applied for a patent.

The first handheld electronic calculator, which performed the four arithmetic functions, measured about six by four by two inches and weighed close to three pounds in its aluminum casing. Texas Instruments did not sell calculators until 1970, when, in collaboration with Canon, it introduced a four-function calculator, the Pocketronic, first in Japan and then in the United States. The Pocketronic was similar in design to the 1967 prototype but weighed only about one pound with its plastic casing and nickel cadmium batteries. As I mentioned earlier, it sold for $400.

In 1970, Gilbert Hyatt filed a patent for the microprocessor (a computer in a single chip), which would further revolutionize the design of computers, large and small, and pave the way for handheld machines with enormous computational power at lower and lower prices. Today, handheld computers can perform all the functions, and more, of the huge computers in use at the University of Wisconsin when I was there in the 1960s. (For its part, the slide rule, after 350 years of steady use, slipped quietly into obscurity within six years of the introduction of the Pocketronic.) And increasingly, these helpful computers are in the hands of clinicians for medical purposes.

The handheld computer in medicine is currently used primarily as a stand-alone machine—as a calculator, of course (for the multiple calculations involved in the day-to-day practice of medicine), as a calendar (for scheduling appointments and meetings), as a reminder (for things to do, such as diagnostic tests to order and treatments to prescribe), as a directory (for street and e-mail addresses and telephone and fax numbers), as a reference (for medically related information, such as medication dosages, toxic side effects, and adverse interactions between drugs), and as an accounting machine (for purposes of billing).

General, encyclopedia-type medical information, such as pharmacological information, is available for electronic transfer to the handheld computer. But to keep track of information specific to an individual patient, a clinician must first enter this information, either manually or by repeatedly downloading from a larger computer, and the process can be cumbersome. (The typewriter-like keyboard, too large for any handheld device, is still the best means for entering free text.) With the rapid development of wireless technology, however, we can expect the handheld computer to be used more and more as an on-line terminal to larger computing systems, including the Internet. This will greatly enhance the power and medical usefulness of these remarkable machines.

We don't tend to think of these machines as part of cybermedicine, and they are not the principal subject of this book. But it is helpful to keep in mind that the most pervasive use of computing technology in medicine to date is the chip in the handheld computer and in the diagnostic machine.

Reporting Results

On the other hand, the results of diagnostic studies generated by machines in the laboratories and clinical departments are still, for the most part, not readily available to the clinicians who need them. Typically, the results are still printed on paper as they are generated and then distributed for use at a later time. In most settings, the doctor must await the distribution of the printed reports, which are known to arrive late and sometimes not at all.

Unfortunately, the use of the computer in direct dialogue with the doctor to communicate the results of diagnostic studies is still more the exception than the rule. Clinician-computer dialogue has a lot of catching up to do. But I get ahead of myself.

CYBERMEDICINE IN TWO TEACHING HOSPITALS

Computers in medicine were still used mostly for financial purposes when, in 1970, I moved from the University of Wisconsin in Madison to join Howard Bleich in the Department of Medicine of the Harvard Medical School in Boston. Howard and I had different clinical interests (he was trained in nephrology, I in neurology), but we shared a common enthusiasm for the use of the computer in medicine.

A New Division

With the invaluable support of Howard Hiatt, who was chairman of Harvard's Department of Medicine at Beth Israel Hospital, Howard Bleich and I wanted to establish a division of clinical computing in the department, analogous to divisions such as cardiology, endocrinology, and gastroenterology. We knew, however, that if we went through administrative channels, there would be only two possible responses. The more likely would be no. The other would be to form a committee—which would still be standing, without resolution, at the end of the century. Accordingly, we took a strip of cardboard, wrote "Division of Clinical Computing" on it, and hung it outside our small cubicle offices. Sometime later the hospital hired sign renovators who advanced through the halls like Costa Rican cutter ants, came across our sign, and promptly replaced it with a metallic plaque firmly ensconced in the concrete siding. We existed de facto! (This can be an effective and perhaps generally applicable strategy, but one that should be used judiciously, maybe once or twice in a lifetime.)

We devoted our efforts during the 1970s to research in cybermedicine, supported by grants from the federal government. Howard studied the use of the computer to interact directly with the doctor to collect, store, and analyze information of diagnostic importance and to offer the doctor advice and suggestions about diagnosis and treatment. I continued my studies of patient-computer dialogue.

In 1976, Howard and I approached the administration of the hospital with a plan to develop, not isolated computer applications for individual departments, but a single, hospital-wide cybermedicine system. Our primary purpose was to use the computer to help doctors, nurses, and other clinicians provide better care for patients. We were convinced, however, that the finances of the hospital would also benefit from the system. At the time, we were most fortunate to have Robert Beckley join our division. Bob went on to provide technical leadership for the project, both at Beth Israel and Brigham and Women's hospitals.

Seven Principles

We had seven principles in mind at the outset—criteria for a successful system that of course are clearer in our minds now, post hoc, than they were when we were getting started.

- *Information should be captured directly at computer terminals located at the point of each transaction, not on pieces of paper.* If information is generated by an automated device, such as a laboratory analyzer, the machine should be connected electronically to the computer, which in turn should help determine the reliability and accuracy of the results. If information must be entered manually, the computer should provide immediate benefit to the person entering this information.

- *Information captured at a terminal or automated device anywhere in the hospital or clinic should be available immediately, if needed, at any other terminal.* Rather than printed reports, which become progressively out of date from the moment they are produced, terminals that provide immediate access to the most up-to-date information should be the principal means of retrieval.

- *The response time of the computer should be rapid.* For the busy physician, nurse, or medical technologist, delays that can be measured in seconds are often unacceptable.

- *The computer should be reliable and accurate.* In the event of failure, the defect should be corrected within minutes, and users should never lose data.

- *Confidentiality should be protected.* Only authorized persons should have access to the data.

- *The computer programs should be friendly to the user and reinforce the user's behavior.* There should be no need for users' manuals. The programs should be self-explanatory.

- *There should be a common registry for all patients.* For each
  patient there should be one and only one set of identifying
  information in the computer, available at all times to authorized
  users and preserved, if possible, in perpetuity. Whenever an
  error in the common database is detected and corrected at any
  terminal, that correction should be immediately available at all
  terminals. The common registry should be shared throughout
  the hospital by all programs that involve identification of a
  patient.

In collaboration with our colleagues in the hospital, we designed,
developed, and installed a hospital-wide cybermedicine system that
we believe fulfilled these criteria, at least for the most part. In the fall
of 1982, on the basis of experience gained at Beth Israel Hospital, we
were asked to develop a similar computing system at Boston's Brigham
and Women's Hospital. Shortly thereafter, we formed the Center for
Clinical Computing (CCC), which was staffed by the highly talented
group of programmers and engineers who had worked with us to
develop the system at Beth Israel, as well as new people who joined us
to work on the system at Brigham and Women's. The development of
the cybermedicine systems for the two hospitals was then under the
direction of the CCC.

In the paragraphs that follow, I will describe these homegrown
systems, which to this day are heavily used and well received by
those who use them. These are certainly not the only hospital-wide
clinical computing systems. Excellent programs such as those at
Duke University, Geneva University, the Kaiser Permanente hospitals in California, LDS Hospital in Salt Lake City, Leiden University
Hospital in the Netherlands, Massachusetts General Hospital in
Boston, Columbia Presbyterian Medical Center, the Regenstrief
Institute in Indianapolis, the University of Missouri, and Vanderbilt University have proved to be highly useful in the practice of
medicine.

The Two Hospitals

Beth Israel Deaconess Medical Center (formed by a merger of Beth
Israel and Deaconess Hospitals in 1996 and a member of Caregroup
Healthcare System) and Brigham and Women's Hospital (a member
of Partners Health Care System) are both teaching hospitals of the
Harvard Medical School. Beth Israel Deaconess has 549 beds, 60

bassinets, and an active emergency room. Each year there are approximately 30,000 admissions and over 500,000 ambulatory (or outpatient) visits. Brigham and Women's Hospital has 716 beds, 96 bassinets, and an active emergency room. Each year there are approximately 40,000 admissions and over 600,000 ambulatory visits. Both hospitals have active teaching programs with medical students, house officers (interns and resident physicians), and clinical fellows (physicians who are training in a medical subspecialty such as cardiology) on every medical and surgical service; and both hospitals have active research programs in each of their academic departments.

The cybermedicine systems were initially developed in Beth Israel and Brigham and Women's hospitals by the staff of the CCC in the MIIS dialect of MUMPS (from Medical Information Technology, Inc.), a pioneering programming language invented by Neil Pappalardo and his colleagues in the 1960s. (If a Nobel Prize for programming languages is ever introduced, Neil Pappalardo would get my vote to be the first recipient.) The programs were run on separate networks of Data General minicomputers, one network at each hospital.

Admitting, Ambulatory, and Medical Records Departments

At both hospitals, the first components of the cybermedicine systems were implemented in the admitting, ambulatory, and medical records departments. These registration programs make up the core of the systems. Although the computer programs were tailored to the individual needs of each hospital, the programs were similar in function. For each of over a million patients cared for at Beth Israel Hospital (now Beth Israel Deaconess) since its system of medical record numbers was established in 1966, and for each of over a million and a half patients at Brigham and Women's Hospital, the name, address, telephone number, social security number, and the names of the parents and spouse are stored in the computers in common registries, a separate one for each hospital.

For the purpose of understanding how the computing works, picture yourself as newly arrived in Boston. You have a new doctor who is on the staff of one of the two hospitals and has referred you there for an appointment. When you arrive as a new patient, whether as an inpatient or an ambulatory patient, a receptionist interviews you and enters your identifying information, in your presence, at a computer terminal. Registration can occur at any of multiple stations throughout the hospitals.

Once your name and other identifying information are in the registry, they stay there indefinitely; thereafter, initiation of a hospital admission, ambulatory visit, or major clinical procedure requires only that someone check and update your information. This is convenient for the receptionist and saves your time as well. It is also more friendly.

If you change your name, address, or other identifying information, corrections can be made, in your presence with your approval, at any terminal by any authorized person who has access to the registry; however, the system preserves an audit trail of the information entered previously, which can be displayed if a question of accuracy arises.

In the admitting departments, staff use terminals for your preadmission (if you are scheduled for hospitalization), to note the time of your arrival, and to keep track of your transfer to different rooms and clinical services when the occasions arise. Unusual circumstances must be accommodated. If you are admitted inadvertently, there is an "unadmit" option; if you are discharged inadvertently, there is an "undischarge" option. Because your current location is known to the computer, meals, mail, medications, laboratory reports, and visitors are all guided correctly to your room.

In the ambulatory departments, staff use terminals to note your arrival and to schedule future visits. The computer applies special rules defined for each clinic to make your appointment; by keeping track of all appointments, it keeps conflicts for both you and your doctor to a minimum. In the operating rooms, staff use terminals to schedule surgical procedures whether you're an inpatient or an ambulatory patient, and to follow your location in the preoperative, operating, and recovery rooms.

Medical Records

In the medical records departments, light pens read bar-coded labels to keep track of your paper chart as it is signed out and returned to the department. (The paper chart, though still in existence, is destined for extinction as records become more fully electronic.) Your chart can be requested from any terminal in either hospital by an authorized person participating in your care. Each request generates a ticket, printed in the medical records department, which provides the last-known location of your chart. Personnel no longer go to shelves jammed with charts only to learn that yours is somewhere else. If you are scheduled to be admitted or seen the next day, the system automatically prints out a request for your chart the night before. If you were to show up in one of the emergency rooms unexpectedly, a request for immediate delivery of your chart would pop out of the printer in the medical records department automatically as soon as the computer received notice of your arrival.

DIAGNOSTIC STUDIES

Once the registration programs were up and running, programs in virtually every laboratory and clinical department were developed and integrated with the registration programs, under the technical and clinical leadership of Gary Horowitz. Consider yourself, if you will, still to be a patient in the hospital.

Laboratories

Computer terminals in the hematology, chemistry, virology, endocrinology, immunology, and microbiology laboratories communicate with the common registry of patients, and your name can be readily located within the registry when you are having laboratory tests performed. When your specimen arrives, such as blood or urine, the technologist identifies you in the registry and indicates which tests have been requested by your doctor. The computer in turn assigns an accession number, notes the date and time, and prints labels and work sheets as required.

In Thomas O'Brien's microbiology laboratory at Brigham and Women's Hospital, where your urine might be cultured for a bacterial infection, there are no printed work sheets. Instead, the computer program, designed by Sandra Goodman and her coworkers, interacts directly with the technologist, presenting each protocol to be followed in a manner individualized for the suspected organisms. If bacteria are cultured from your urine, their descriptions, together with their sensitivities to antimicrobial agents that could be used for your treatment, are entered directly at the terminals at the time the results are determined; these data are then available to your doctor upon request from any terminal in the system. (Terminals are scattered throughout the hospital, in the ambulatory clinics, and in the doctors' offices.)

Automated devices in the laboratories connect to the computer networks electronically. Results of studies obtained with these devices, such as your blood count and blood sugar, are first displayed on terminals in the laboratories, where a technologist checks them. If you have had a blood count in the recent past, the results of that count appear next to the current ones; on occasion, a marked disparity between a recent and current result has enabled the technologist to detect a mislabeled specimen or the effect of an interfering substance causing an error in the test. If the results of your test are markedly abnormal or the current result is substantially different from the previous determination, the computer automatically flags the results; such results would then be rechecked by a senior technologist and telephoned to your doctor at the number provided by the computer. In this way, the computer helps to ensure the quality of tests performed. Once verified, the results of your tests are released for viewing by your doctor at any terminal.

Clinical Departments

Cardiology, neurology, radiology, and pathology are representative of departments that have been computerized. In the exercise, echocardiography, and cardiac catheterization laboratories of the cardiology department, the technologist would use the computer to identify you in the registry and to indicate the procedure to be performed. The results of your study—a cardiac catheterization, for example—would then be recorded at a terminal and approved by a staff cardiologist. Before the computer system was in place, weeks or sometimes months might pass before your results would find their way to your chart; results are now available within a few days, both for viewing on terminals and for placement in your paper chart.

If an electrocardiogram is indicated at Beth Israel Deaconess, your doctor uses one of the ubiquitous terminals to request the study. Your identifying information is then electronically transferred to the electrocardiography chart for use at the time of your study. Once the results have been approved, they are transferred electronically to the hospital's computers, which make the verbal report (with the electrocardiogram tracing itself if your doctor is using a PC) available for viewing.

In the neurology department at Beth Israel Deaconess, technologists in the electroencephalography and electromyography laboratories can use the computer to identify you in the registry, to indicate the study to be performed, and to record the results of your study, which are then approved by a staff neurologist and made available for viewing on the hospital's terminals.

And so it is in radiology. When you are about to have a chest X ray at Beth Israel Deaconess, the receptionist identifies you at a terminal and denotes the examination. The computer then prints a work card for the technologist, a label for the new film jacket, a transportation ticket that provides your room number (if you are hospitalized), and an identification card that is optically photographed to label the new films at the time of the X-ray exposure. At the same time, a printer located in the file room produces a request to retrieve your previous films.

When the technologist indicates at a terminal that your examination has been completed, the computer automatically adds the charge for your films to your hospital bill—a function more in the hospital's interest than yours. As your films (the front and side views) emerge from the dryer, they are merged with any earlier films you may have had and presented to your radiologist for interpretation and side-by-side comparison; looking for changes over time is an important aspect of diagnostic radiology. The radiologist could then record the diagnostic interpretation directly at a terminal with an interactive coding system developed in the radiology department by Morris Simon, Brian Leeming, Jerry Jackson, and their coworkers. (Some radiologists prefer to dictate their reports, which are then transcribed into a word processor that is part of the same computing system.) Your radiologist would then use the terminal to edit and approve the report, which would then be released for viewing by authorized clinicians in patient care areas throughout the hospital and clinics.

In the surgical pathology departments in the two hospitals, where biopsy specimens are examined, and the cytology departments, where Pap tests are performed, every specimen is registered in the computer; if you have had specimens analyzed previously, the program provides the identification numbers so that the slides can be retrieved and reexamined under the microscope. Anatomical and microscopical descriptions of each new specimen are transcribed into a word processor in the computer. The pathologist then reviews and edits this report at any available terminal, and as with all the diagnostic studies, releases the report for viewing on terminals throughout the hospitals and ambulatory facilities.

Programs in virtually every laboratory and department devoted to treatment have also been developed and integrated with the registration systems. The blood banks and the pharmacies are two examples.

BLOOD BANK. In the blood banks, where donated blood is stored and distributed for use in transfusions, the programs maintain crucial information in case you should need a blood transfusion. This includes your transfusion history—Have you ever had one? Have you ever had a problem with a transfusion?—your blood type and associated antibodies, and any specific requirements you might have, such as the need for blood that has been irradiated or is low in white blood cells. If you are about to have surgery, this information is automatically transmitted to the blood bank from the program that scheduled your operating room.

The terminals are also used to maintain an inventory of blood that is available for use. When your doctor requests blood for you, the computer helps find the most appropriate units, looking first for autologous blood (that is, your own previously donated blood), then for blood that has been cross-matched and held in reserve for you, and finally for blood that is most likely to be suitable for you on the basis of your type, the antibodies in your blood, and any specific requirements you might have.

PHARMACY. As designed by Richard Pope in the early days of the CCC system, the pharmacy computing system serves an important role. At each hospital, the computers maintain the formularies—the lists of available medications. If your doctor requests medications for you while you are in the hospital, the computer helps to organize the preparation and distribution of your medications, whether they are to be taken by mouth or intravenously. A list of each of your medications is then made available for viewing on terminals throughout the hospital. The computers also assist with inventory by permitting surveillance of available medications, both according to manufacturer and according to functional class.

FINANCIAL COMPUTING

Virtually every one of the services you receive, whether it is your ambulatory visit, inpatient admission, diagnostic study, medication order, or blood transfusion, must be registered in the computer before it can be performed. Manual registration and identification procedures that were once used throughout the hospitals—procedures that were fraught with error and lost charges—have largely disappeared. After the service has been performed and its results have been recorded in the computer, the charge is automatically added to your file. In this way, more than 90 percent of the charges are obtained as a by-product of the cybermedicine systems.

At Beth Israel Deaconess, these charges are transferred by magnetic tape each day to the hospital's fiscal computing system (in a separate facility not in the CCC network), which prints the bills and performs other financial operations.

At Brigham and Women's Hospital, where the financial programs were developed as part of the CCC cybermedicine system by Edna Moody and her colleagues, the billing office was integrated with the clinical computing network. The programs produce billing tapes for both inpatients and ambulatory patients, and the tapes are transferred to third-party payers such as Medicare, Medicaid, and Blue Cross. In turn, remittance tapes from third-party payers, which accompany the payment checks, are read by the computer and used to match the payment received with your account.

Other financial programs on Brigham and Women's network include a general ledger program that accumulates financial data needed for managers; a purchasing program that maintains an inventory of supplies, keeps track of vendors, and computes the amount owed to the hospital's suppliers; and a personnel program that stores data regarding employees and computes their paychecks.

At each hospital, Karen Franklin and her colleagues developed programs to assign a diagnosis-related group (DRG) to each patient and to alert the medical records department when additional coding may entitle the hospital to increased reimbursement. At Beth Israel Deaconess, the computer prints reminders listing the abnormal laboratory results of patients on Medicare that may entitle the hospital to additional reimbursement.

It is important to keep in mind, however, that when third parties such as the government, managed care agencies, and insurance companies pay the medical bills, they ask for clinical information to justify the payments. This creates a breach in the confidential relationship between you and your doctor. But this is the topic of a later chapter.

—◇◇◇—

The ultimate goal of hospital computing is to improve patient care. Sometimes this gets forgotten. Sometimes the computing in an individual department becomes an end in itself, independent of the collective goal of patient care. The goal in the clinical laboratory is not to have a well-run laboratory in isolation from the rest of the hospital; the goal is to get the results of diagnostic studies to the doctor, with accuracy and reliability. The goal in finance is not to make money; the goal is to support good medical care.

In most hospitals and clinics to this day, the computing is mostly financial, under the auspices of the chief financial officer, and managerial, under the auspices of a chief information officer. The acronym MIS stands for *Management* Information Systems, not *Medical*. It is my abiding hope that the "M" in MIS will soon stand for "Medical."

When the "M" does stand for "Medical," what will this mean for the doctor?

FROM THE CYBERHERO COLLECTION...

BUGMAN

- ANALYZES EXCRETION ROUTES IN A SINGLE BYTE!
- LISTS ANTIBIOTIC EFFECTIVENESS FASTER THAN A SPEEDING BULLET!
- DOSAGE GUIDELINES MORE POWERFUL THAN A LOCOMOTIVE!

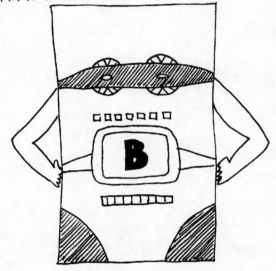

CHAPTER SEVEN

Cybermedicine in the Care of the Patient

S ince the inception of the CCC cybermedicine systems at Beth Israel and Brigham and Women's hospitals, physicians, nurses, medical students, and other authorized clinicians have gained access by going to any terminal (or personal computer serving as a terminal in the network), pressing the "Enter" key, and typing a confidential password. The CCC system then offers clinicians important demographic information, the results of diagnostic studies, help in the day-to-day practice of medicine, help with decisions, and help with communication. Picture yourself once again as a patient in the hospital. Your doctor is on the staff and has a password granting her (let me assume henceforth that your doctor is a woman) access to the programs.

THE COMPUTER AS A CLINICIAN'S ASSISTANT

Clinical information about you as a patient is retrieved through Patient Lookup, the most heavily used option in the CCC system. To use Patient Lookup, your doctor must first identify you by entering your name—or your medical record number, your financial number, your social security number, your room number, or the name of the nursing station nearest you, such as "coronary care unit." We have worked hard to make it easy for your doctor to find you. The computer adjusts for misspellings; our clinicians spell with admirable creativity.

Once your doctor has located you, the computer asks why she wants access to your electronic record, whether it is for clinical care, research, teaching, or administrative purposes. This information can then be helpful in evaluating the various ways in which the programs are used and the appropriateness of their use.

The computer then displays a list of options that can provide your doctor with needed information about you.

Demographic Information

If your doctor selects the Demographics/Discharge Diagnoses option, the computer displays your demographic information from the common registry; it then lists the names of the doctors who saw you for ambulatory appointments, your visits to the emergency room, and your previous hospital admissions together with your diagnoses for each admission.

Results of Diagnostic Studies

The computer then displays a list of laboratories and departments from which your doctor can view the results of laboratory tests and clinical procedures. Suppose your doctor chooses All Labs—Most Recent Results. The computer will then display all your results for the past two days if you are an inpatient, or all results since your most recent admission or visit to a clinic if you are an ambulatory patient. Alternatively, your doctor can specify any date range or any particular department or laboratory. Information from the laboratories is available as soon as the diagnostic studies have been performed. Results are displayed in reverse chronological order, with the most recent results first. To assist your physician in planning her course of action, abnormal values are tagged as such, and results that might require immediate attention are further denoted.

If your doctor chooses Cardiology, Cytology, Neurophysiology, Radiology, or Surgical Pathology, the computer displays the examinations performed and a summary of the findings and their diagnostic interpretations; if she chooses Operating Room History/Recovery Room, the computer displays your surgical procedures, either scheduled or already performed; if she chooses Blood Bank, the computer displays your blood type and associated antibodies, your transfusion history (including any adverse reactions), and an inventory of cross-matched blood (or autologous blood if you have donated any) that is held in reserve and ready for her to use; and if she chooses Pharmacy, the computer offers her options to view the medications used during your hospitalization—either current medications or a summary for the present or most recent admission—and problems you might have had when taking your medications.

Most of this information is available from the terminals for ten years; after that your information is removed from the active disk files but kept on magnetic tape for use if a retrospective analysis is needed.

Help in the Day-to-Day Practice of Medicine

The following options help your doctor with the daily routines of your care. The computers maintain a Personal Patient List—a list of the patients under her care. When you are admitted to the hospital, your name is automatically placed on your doctor's list.

With Edit Personal Patient List, your doctor and nurse can add or delete names from their lists. With View Hospitalized Patient List, your doctor can view the names of patients who are on her list and are currently in the hospital or have been seen by her that day in the emergency room. With Personal Patient Lookup, your doctor can step through the clinical data on each of her hospitalized or ambulatory patients without having to enter the names. This option can remind your doctor about laboratory tests that have been ordered. A Cross Coverage option permits your doctor, when she is temporarily off duty, to authorize others to look at information they may need to care for her patients. And at Beth Israel Deaconess, a Discharge Summary program, developed by Daniel Sands and his colleagues in the CCC, helps your doctor coordinate each patient's clinical information for use at the time of discharge from the hospital.

The training programs for house officers in teaching hospitals are stressful, and these young doctors sometimes experience symptoms of anxiety and depression. At Beth Israel Deaconess, an option called Confidential Counseling for House Officers gives the names, telephone numbers, and page numbers of clinicians in the Department of Psychiatry who are available to help house officers in distress (in the strictest of confidence). Further options permit your doctor to order tests and procedures, request delivery of your paper chart, and review the Medical Executive Committee's recommended preoperative evaluation procedures (as a check for good patient care before surgery).

A Universal Precautions option at Beth Israel Deaconess offers your doctor a teaching program on safety measures when handling blood and other fluids from patients. Developed by Tamar Barlam, Dori Zaleznik, and their colleagues in the Division of Infectious Diseases, together with Hollis Kowaloff and her colleagues in the CCC, this program is designed to help prevent untoward events, for example, an accidental needle stick, that could result in transmission of a viral infection such as AIDS or hepatitis. The program will also advise your doctor about the appropriate procedures to follow if an accident occurs.

With Notes, your doctor can type a message about your medical care that will be displayed on the Personal Patient Lookup screen. These notes, which become part of your clinical record, can be used to remind her about specific problems such as an adverse reaction to an antibiotic or an allergy to a radiographic dye used in certain X-ray studies. Incomplete Medical Record informs your doctor about administrative chores that need to be done—discharge summaries that need to be dictated and medical records that need to be signed. (This is the least popular of the ancillary options.)

Utility opens up a set of programs to assist your doctor. One of them allows her to change her password in case of a suspected breach in security. An option labeled How To Use The Computer Terminal offers instructions for newcomers to the system and reminders for more experienced users. (When an option is confusing, typing a question mark typically results in an explanation.) A Telephone Directory provides the phone number, beeper number, and room number of each member of the staff and of each department, as well as the weekly schedule of physicians in their specialty clinics. A Doctor's Office directory provides the address, phone number, and specialty (at Brigham and Women's Hospital) of each staff physician. This program helps house officers contact attending physicians whose offices are outside the hospital.

Help in the Ambulatory Setting

Charles Safran, David Rind, Daniel Sands, and their colleagues in the CCC and Health Care Associates at Beth Israel Deaconess have developed numerous programs, as part of the hospital-wide cybermedicine system, that are specifically designed to help clinicians in the ambulatory setting. Virtually all of the narrative generated by your doctor becomes part of your electronic record, either by direct entry by her at her computer terminal or by transcription of her dictated notes and letters. This includes prescriptions for medications as well as any allergic reactions to medications should they occur. This narrative information, together with the comprehensive set of information from the laboratories and clinical departments, is then available to her from any of the cybermedicine terminals at any time of day or night. Among the many options now available to your doctor and her colleagues is a program that will display her appointment schedule for the day. For each patient scheduled, the computer presents a list of past and current medical problems (in keeping with the problem-oriented medical record, based on the pioneering contribution of Lawrence Weed) and an electronically stored narrative for each problem. The summary includes a list of the patient's medications and a list of appointments with other consulting physicians. This enables your doctor to refresh her memory and make plans for the future. By recent count, over a thousand physicians and nurses use the cybermedicine system in the ambulatory setting.

Help for the Nurses

Nurses are among the most frequent users of the many options in the CCC system. Some of these options, developed with Joyce Clifford, Patricia Bourie, Radene Chapman, Peggy Reiley, and their colleagues at Beth Israel Hospital, were designed specifically for nurses to use in patient care. These include Automated Nursing Assessment, which helps nurses assess the overall clinical situation of each patient, with specific nursing needs in mind; Bulletin Board, which displays standards of care and clinical guidelines; Dietary Orders, which allows nurses to request meals with specific clinical needs in mind; and Surgery Scheduling, which displays the operating room schedule and helps nurses get patients ready for surgery.

Help with Decisions

Also available at the two hospitals are programs designed to help your doctor provide you with better medical care as well as to help her or other doctors conduct research of potential benefit to patients in the future. Such programs are sometimes called "expert systems," but we prefer to refer to them as decision-support programs or computer-based consultation. Many such programs, developed with the technical support of Elaine Bianco and her coworkers, are in use at both hospitals. The following consultation programs are available to all authorized clinicians at Beth Israel Deaconess.

ACID-BASE CONSULTATION. If your doctor needs help in deciding about intravenous fluids, she can use an electrolyte and acid-base program that automatically obtains laboratory data such as your serum sodium concentration, serum creatinine concentration, and blood pH from the hospital's computer network. It then directs a dialogue in which your doctor supplies clinical information, such as your weight and any evidence of congestive heart failure. On the basis of the abnormalities detected, the program then asks further questions as needed to characterize the electrolyte and acid-base disturbances. Upon completion of the interchange, the program produces an evaluation note that resembles a consultant's discussion of the problem. The note includes a list of diagnostic possibilities, an explanation of the pathophysiology, recommendations for therapy, suggestions for additional laboratory studies, precautionary measures indicated by the illness or its treatment, and references to the medical literature. Originally developed by Howard Bleich in 1968, this was to my knowledge the first computing program to offer consultation on how best to treat a medical problem.

TREATING INFECTIOUS DISEASES. This program, which we call Bugman, provides your doctor with an interactive guide to the diagnosis and treatment of infectious diseases. Originally written in Converse by Michael Bookman, Bugman provides such information as the mechanism of action, route of excretion (such as the urine), and duration of effectiveness of antibiotics in the hospital's formulary. The program also lists the relative effectiveness of various antibiotics against various pathogenic bacteria, and provides dosage guidelines and cost comparisons for each antibiotic. A similar program written in Converse by Richard Platt—Antibiotic Information—provides clinicians at Brigham and Women's Hospital with guidance in the use of antimicrobial agents.

AN ON-LINE REFERENCE BOOK FOR MEDICATIONS. This program is an on-line version of the *Physicians' Desk Reference* (PDR). The book's indexes for generic name, brand name, product category, and company name have been merged. When your doctor enters the name of a medication, the program offers information about its pharmacology and the indications for its use, together with its side effects, interactions with other drugs, and dosage. Perhaps as a reflection of our times, clinicians have requested information about fluoxetine (Prozac), which is used for depression, more often than about any other medication.

MEDICATIONS IN THE PHARMACY. Also written in Converse, Drugman is an interactive hospital formulary. The pharmacy maintains information about new drugs, new treatments such as calcium supplementation, and drugs being studied. Unlike the information in the on-line PDR, which is gathered from the manufacturers, the information in Drugman is gathered by a staff pharmacist in the hospital and reviewed by a senior staff physician before being released for viewing on your doctor's CCC terminal. Drugman contains data on indications for use, dosage, pharmacology, adverse drug reactions, and cost, and it compares medications in terms of cost-effectiveness.

DRUG INFORMATION. This program offers information about the costs of medications. This helps your doctor choose the least expensive medication from among those of the same quality.

A PROGRAM FOR PATIENTS WITH AIDS. HIV ProtoCall, also written in Converse, was developed in collaboration with the AIDS Clinical Trials Group of the hospital. It advises your doctor on the availability of experimental protocols for patients with HIV infection and on the care of patients taking experimental drugs. With HIV ProtoCall, your doctor can quickly learn whether her patients meet the criteria for inclusion in treatment protocols at any of the treatment centers in the Boston area.

WITHDRAWAL OF THERAPY. This program offers guidelines for withdrawing or limiting the use of life-sustaining measures when death is close at hand and pain and suffering are to be avoided. The guidelines, which first and foremost respect the wishes of the patient and family but also conform to hospital policy and state laws, are available to help the clinician at any time of day or night from any of the terminals.

ADDITIONAL HELP WITH DECISIONS. Also available under the decision support options at Beth Israel Deaconess is a program developed by Daniel Sands that offers the solutions to a number of mathematical formulas. These are formulas that are used routinely in the care of very sick patients but that most clinicians do not know by heart. And in the ambulatory setting, a program developed by Jonathan Einbinder and his colleagues in the CCC would advise your doctor on the use of anticoagulants to prevent the formation of blood clots. This may be necessary in patients with artificial heart valves or thrombophlebitis.

Jogging the Memory On-Line

My father, a nuclear physicist, shared my concern about the exaggerated emphasis in medicine on memorization. He noticed that doctors seemed embarrassed when they had to look something up, whereas physical scientists would rely unabashedly on printed material for data and formulas, including their own. He thought it would be better for patients if doctors could come to grips with the imperfections of the human mind and rely more heavily on reference material and other reminders, even when they were confident of their information.

Fortunately, the excessive reliance on memory among physicians has begun to wane, with the help of the computer, and two physicians and their colleagues deserve a sizable share of the credit. Homer Warner and his colleagues at the LDS Hospital in Salt Lake City pioneered the development of the HELP system, which has proved to be highly effective in helping clinicians with clinical decisions and reminding them of important medical matters that need attention. And, in another pioneering effort, Clement McDonald and his colleagues at the University of Indiana showed that errors in diagnosis and treatment could be reduced significantly when physicians were presented with computer-generated reminders. Furthermore, they discovered that the impact of the reminders was independent of the level of the physician's training. Senior residents in their study benefited as much from the reminders as did interns. In fact, the reminders had their greatest effect on a second-year resident, even though he had insisted at the beginning of the study that "what was needed was education of bad physicians about what they did not know, not reminders to good physicians about what they knew."

Alerts and Reminders

More recently, Charles Safran, David Rind, and coworkers in the CCC at Beth Israel Deaconess Medical Center have differentiated between an *alert,* which they define as a warning of a clinical event that needs immediate attention, and a *reminder,* which they define as an event that should be attended to in conjunction with the routine care of the patient. With the CCC system, the entire hospital and all its clinics and ambulatory offices share one common database of patients. All the information from the laboratories and clinical departments for each patient is available to authorized clinicians on all the terminals. This enables your doctor to see alerts and reminders about a wide variety of medical issues whenever she signs on at a terminal.

One use of alerts pertains to kidney function. Many medications in current use are either excreted by the kidneys after acting therapeutically, or potentially toxic to the kidneys during their therapeutic action. If you are on a drug such as cimetidine (for peptic ulcers) that is excreted by the kidneys and your kidneys are not functioning properly, the level of the drug in your bloodstream may become unacceptably high. If you are taking a medication such as gentamicin (a powerful antibiotic for use against life-threatening infections), it may damage your kidneys. In either case, it would be wise for your doctor to consider reducing the dose or switching to a different drug.

The best laboratory measure of kidney function is the serum level of creatinine, a product of muscle metabolism that the kidneys normally excrete from the plasma into the urine. An abnormally high serum creatinine may indicate impaired kidney function. At Beth Israel Deaconess Medical Center, if you are a hospitalized patient whose serum creatinine is high and you are taking either cimetidine or gentamicin (or a drug with similar effects on the kidneys), an alert would go out automatically from the computer to your doctor the next time she signs on to the computer. As another example, for patients with AIDS, an alert goes out automatically when it is time for an important diagnostic test or a change in treatment.

Reminders, on the other hand, are invoked primarily in the ambulatory setting. When your doctor signs on at the CCC system in anticipation of your visit, she is reminded of the timing of such important procedures as an influenza vaccination, a Pap test, or a tetanus shot.

The Quest for Additional Information

When your doctor makes "rounds" in the hospital (meaning that she visits patients with interns, residents, and medical students), she tends to refer to two sources of information for help with problems that come up: the medical library and past clinical experience. "I think there was an article about this in the *New England Journal of Medicine*," and "I once saw a patient with a similar medical problem," are commonly heard comments along clinical corridors. Two programs conceived and developed by members of the CCC were designed to jog your doctor's memory and to help her to become better informed—PaperChase and ClinQuery.

SEARCHING THE MEDICAL LITERATURE. PaperChase, the bibliographic retrieval program mentioned in Chapter Five, permits your doctor to search the National Library of Medicine's database of references to the medical literature (MEDLINE). She can perform a search, read summaries, and—at a cost of $12 per article—order mailed photocopies of the full text. PaperChase provides access to over nine million references to articles in forty-three hundred journals dating back to 1966. But more of PaperChase a little later.

SEARCHING THE CLINICAL DATABASE. Patterned after PaperChase and developed under the direction of Charles Safran, ClinQuery is a program on the CCC system that retrieves clinical information and enables clinicians and clinical investigators to search the computerized clinical data of all patients admitted to Beth Israel Hospital since 1984, and Beth Israel Deaconess Medical Center subsequent to the merger (491,797 admissions through December 2000). Lists of patients based on demographic information; on results of diagnostic studies from the surgical pathology, cardiology, radiology, and clinical laboratories; and on blood transfusions, medications, and discharge diagnoses (from medicine, surgery, and all other clinical services) can be used to identify patients with attributes of particular interest.

ClinQuery has two primary uses: patient care and clinical research. If your doctor is deciding how best to care for you, she can use Clin-Query to look for a list of patients with a similar problem, and then examine each of these patients' medical records to look for treatments that might help you as well. If your doctor is doing research and has an interest, for example, in reasons for return visits to the emergency room, she can use ClinQuery to make lists of patients who have been seen in the emergency room and use the lists to explore alternative hypotheses. To protect patients' confidentiality, names and other personally identifying information are not displayed in conjunction with the lists of patients retrieved with ClinQuery.

Help with Communication

E-mail—now a generic term—is also the name of a system developed by Robert Beckley, Saul Bloom, Howard Bleich, and our colleagues in the CCC that was perhaps the first such communication system to be installed in a clinical facility (at Beth Israel Hospital in the late 1970s and at Brigham and Women's Hospital in 1983). It permits your doctor to send and receive messages from any of the terminals located throughout the hospitals and clinics. Our homegrown e-mail system has been the cybermedicine lifeline, greatly enhancing and actually humanizing communication within the walls of our hospitals and now with the outside world over the Internet. But more about e-mail for the clinician shortly.

NEW DIRECTIONS

In 1989, upon completion of the CCC cybermedicine project at Brigham and Women's Hospital, administrative responsibility for computing was transferred to the hospital. Since that time, clinicians, computer scientists, and programmers there have developed a number of new programs to help clinicians in the care of their patients. David Bates, Gilad Kuperman, Jonathan Teich, and their colleagues have incorporated into the hospital-wide computing system programs that enable a physician to enter requests both for diagnostic studies such as laboratory tests and for therapeutic regimens such as medication orders, and then alert the physician to possible problems with the studies requested and treatments proposed. The programs will then suggest alternative approaches, when appropriate, and, further, will alert the physician to the need for rapid intervention when a patient is found to have markedly abnormal laboratory results.

In 1996, administrative responsibility for the CCC cybermedicine system at Beth Israel Deaconess Medical Center was transferred to the medical center. Computing systems are now being converted to new machines and computer programming languages and more and more use is being made of Web technology. The new technology should provide more modern visual presentation to the user, together with increased speed and efficiency. There are now over eight thousand computer terminals, including PCs being used as terminals, at Beth Israel Deaconess Medical Center—and well over ten thousand terminals at Brigham and Women's Hospital and their related clinics and private offices.

On the other hand, my colleagues at the two hospitals and in the CCC prefer to have cybermedicine systems judged on the basis of how well they work, how useful they are, and how frugally they run. In these days of computing glitz, where the computer culturati flaunt their jargon with an Orwellian facileness (try *open systems, data warehouse,* and *connectivity* for starters), where new computing and new words to describe it (for example, *best of breed*) are considered desirable solely because they are new even when their computing is outperformed by the old (*legacy system* in the newest computerspeak), it is helpful to ask the old question, "What is the problem we are trying to solve?"

The problem we are trying to solve with computing for the clinician is a problem in communication—the current insufficiency of readily available information that could help clinicians care for patients. If the computer can be programmed to communicate with the doctor, at his or her beck and call, to provide the results of diagnostic studies, offer advice and consultation, and give access to articles in medical journals, the doctor and patient will be well served even if the technology behind the computer terminal is behind the times. The patient in pain is less interested in three-dimensional color graphics than in competent care.

It is not sufficient for those of us working in the field of cybermedicine to develop such systems, install them, and then proclaim success. Rather, it is incumbent on us to do our best to evaluate the impact of our efforts, for good or for bad, on the practice of medicine. All too often, programs purporting to do clinical computing are touted and marketed in the absence of evidence about their quality and usefulness. Questions such as "How often do the doctors use your system?" tend to go unanswered.

Let us turn, then, to a look at the CCC cybermedicine system in use.

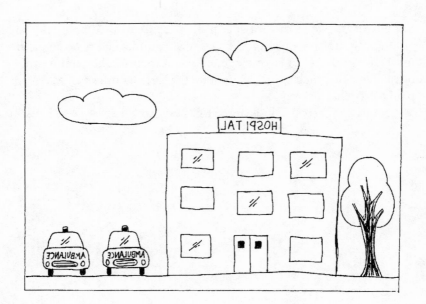

CHAPTER EIGHT

How Well Does It Work?

Y ears ago, John Watson and B. F. Skinner taught that behavior is shaped by its consequences. If the consequences are reinforcing, the behavior is strengthened. If not, the behavior tends to disappear. Thus physicians and other clinicians will interact with computers if the interaction is helpful. It has been our working premise over the years that clinicians will be ardent users of computing systems if the systems are useful in the practice of medicine. If going on-line assists in the day-to-day activities of an arduous clinical practice, the doctor will go on-line early and often. If the computer makes it easier to get the results of diagnostic studies, if it helps with time-consuming administrative chores, if it offers good advice and consultation, if it offers ready access to the medical literature, and if it helps the doctor communicate with others in the field, these services will be in great demand. But how do we go about testing this premise?

ASSESSING THE CLINICIAN'S USE

At Beth Israel Deaconess Medical Center and Brigham and Women's Hospital, we have done our best to evaluate the usefulness of the CCC cybermedicine system. We have tried to address six specific questions, namely intensity of use, attitude of users, effect on quality of patient care, educational value, financial impact, and cost:

- *How often does the voluntary user—the clinician who is under no obligation to do so—use cybermedicine?* There is no a priori reason for the clinician to use a computer unless it offers information that cannot be obtained as readily somewhere else.

- *What is the attitude of the users toward cybermedicine?* Do they perceive it to be helpful?

- *What is the effect of cybermedicine on the quality of medical care?* This, of course is our reason for being.

- *What is the effect of cybermedicine on the education of clinicians?* Does the computing help or hinder the learning process?

- *What is the effect of cybermedicine on the finances of the hospital or clinic?* Does the computing help out in the financial department?

- *What is the cost of cybermedicine?* Is good cybermedicine affordable?

To expand on the first point, the results of diagnostic studies are typically available in printed reports; educational information and consultation can be obtained from books, journals, and personal communication; and many of the references to the medical literature can be found in a book from the National Library of Medicine, the *Index Medicus.* If a computer purported to perform these functions is seldom used, it probably offers no advantage over traditional methods of processing and presenting this available information. Attention should then be directed to the program rather than the clinician.

VOLUNTARY USE OF CYBERMEDICINE

A distinguishing feature of the cybermedicine systems at Beth Israel Deaconess Medical Center and Brigham and Women's Hospital is the intensity and extensiveness of their use, without coercion. Doctors, nurses, medical students, and other clinicians are heavy users of the CCC system. As they have learned that the programs are reliable and that the computers are almost never down, they have come to rely on the computing system for help in the care of patients. When the laboratory programs were first available at Beth Israel Hospital (before terminals were installed on nursing units), house officers discovered that they could see the results on terminals in the laboratories as soon as the tests had been performed. They descended from the nursing stations and commandeered the laboratory terminals, sometimes to the consternation of the technologists. In response to the demands of the house officers, terminals were installed on the nursing stations throughout the hospital and used with increasing frequency.

Keeping Track of Use

The computer-assigned passwords that identify each user and permit access to the CCC system also provide an electronic signature for each transaction with the computer. We have used these signatures to determine the frequency with which the computer programs are used by staff doctors, house officers, clinical fellows, nurses, medical students, and other clinicians in the two hospitals. The intensity of the use by these voluntary users can be taken as a measure of the system's helpfulness.

Use at Beth Israel Deaconess Medical Center

During the week of April 6 to 12, 1984, 818 clinicians at Beth Israel Hospital (staff physicians, nurses, clinical fellows, house officers, medical students, and health assistants) used the patient lookup option 16,768 times. They looked up information on hospitalized patients 12,688 times and information on ambulatory patients 4,080 times. The daily census averaged 455 patients; information on each hospitalized patient was looked up an average of four times per day.

Over the next four years, use increased dramatically. During the week of October 3 to 9, 1988, a total of 1,737 clinicians—232 staff physicians, 893 nurses, 64 clinical fellows, 236 house officers, 59 medical students, and 253 health assistants—used one or more of the patient care options 58,757 times. The patient lookup option was the most heavily used. During that week, 1,436 clinicians looked up data on 900 hospitalized patients 27,729 times—a 218 percent increase over the counting in 1984. During that same week, 1,045 clinicians looked up clinical data on 4,379 ambulatory patients 13,229 times—an increase of 324 percent since 1984. As would be expected in a teaching hospital, clinicians in training were the heaviest users, looking up clinical data 15,728 times, with a mean of 54 lookups per intern and resident and 49 per medical student.

Use continued to increase. During the week of February 23 to 29, 1992, a total of 2,354 clinicians—352 staff physicians, 1,022 nurses, 103 clinical fellows, 305 house officers, 49 medical students, and 523 health assistants—used one or more of the options in the cybermedicine system 69,784 times. The Patient Lookup option continued to be the most heavily used. During that week, clinicians looked up data on hospitalized patients 34,614 times—a 272 percent increase over a comparable period in 1984, during the early days of the CCC system. During the same week, clinicians looked up clinical data on ambulatory patients 21,497 times—an increase of 526 percent since 1984. As would be expected in a teaching hospital, clinicians in training were the heaviest users of Patient Lookup, with a mean of 45 inquiries per house officer and 25 lookups per medical student.

During the week of April 25 to May 1, 1994, the number of lookups of clinical information for inpatients was down to 30,264, well below the comparable week in 1992. On the other hand, the number of lookups for ambulatory patients was up to 27,023, an indication of the shift in American medicine to ambulatory care. And during the week of April 27 to May 3, 1998, the number of lookups for inpatients was up to 35,229, and the number of lookups for ambulatory patients was up to 44,383. The option used most frequently (27,062 times) was All Labs Most Recent Results, which as I've said provides recent results from all laboratories and clinical departments. Since we counted each use of this option as a single inquiry, the reported number understates by a wide margin the number of contacts with laboratories and clinical departments that would have been required to provide the same information.

The programs designed to help with decisions have also been used with increasing frequency. During the week in 1992 PaperChase was used to perform 1,556 searches of the National Library of Medicine's MEDLINE database, and clinicians used the other decision-support programs a total of 1,288 times. During the comparable week in 1998, PaperChase was used to perform 1,794 searches, and clinicians used the other decision-support programs over 4,000 times. In addition, over 30,000 messages were sent by e-mail.

Subsequent to the merger between Beth Israel and Deaconess hospitals in 1996, the CCC cybermedicine system was extended to the Deaconess Hospital facility and, since 1998, the voluntary use of the system throughout Beth Israel Deaconess Medical Center has continued to increase. During the week of September 18 to 24, 2000, clinicians used the patient care options 114,891 times. (As I mentioned, more than eight thousand terminals are deployed throughout the medical center.) As I write, there are 1,034 staff physicians, 1,983 nurses, 258 clinical fellows, 630 house officers, and 395 medical students with passwords to the CCC cybermedicine system at Beth Israel Deaconess Medical Center.

Use at Brigham and Women's Hospital

At Brigham and Women's Hospital, use of the CCC cybermedicine system has been equally intensive. During the week of October 3 to 9, 1988, 2,262 clinicians at Brigham and Women's Hospital—549 physicians and 1,713 nurses, health assistants, and students—used one or more of the options in the clinical information system 89,101 times. As at Beth Israel Hospital, Patient Lookup was used most often: clinicians made inquires about 1,306 inpatients 40,998 times and about 5,402 ambulatory patients 14,383 times, and physicians in training were the heaviest users. Among the 299 house officers who used the system during that week, the mean number of inquiries was 59.

During the same week in October 1988, clinicians used the consultation program on antibiotics 111 times and used PaperChase to perform 947 searches of the medical literature.

Since 1988, in conjunction with an increasing number of terminals and their ready accessibility (now over ten thousand), use at Brigham and Women's Hospital has continued to rise. As I write, the cybermedicine systems at Brigham and Women's Hospital and Beth Israel Deaconess Medical Center are among the most heavily used systems in the world.

ATTITUDE OF THE USER

In 1982, I wrote a computer-administered interview to find out how the clinicians at Beth Israel Hospital felt about the CCC cybermedicine system. Written in Converse, the interview asked the users to rate the computer's helpfulness, efficiency, and ease of use, and then requested comments and suggestions.

The interview was incorporated into the sign-on procedure; on entering a password, each qualified user was given the opportunity to answer the questions immediately, to defer them until a later date, or to avoid them altogether. Those who deferred were again invited to participate after a delay of at least twenty-four hours. Those who refused were asked to reconsider after a delay of at least a week. Those who refused twice were not asked again.

The results were gratifying. Of the 1,429 people invited to respond to the computer-based interview, 79 percent agreed, and both obligatory users (those such as departmental and laboratory personnel whose jobs required them to work at terminals) and voluntary users (the clinicians who could have used more traditional means of communication if they so desired) praised the computing system. Of the 545 obligatory users—the inpatient admitting officers, medical record administrators, and laboratory technologists—over 70 percent indicated that the computer had made their work more accurate, easier, faster, and more interesting. Of the 586 clinicians who completed the survey, over 80 percent indicated that they used the computer terminals "most of the time" to look up laboratory results and found the computer terminals "very helpful" in doing so. Staff physicians, interns, residents, medical students, and nurses were similar in their estimates for the helpfulness of the computer.

At the end of the survey, users were asked to comment, if they wished, on their reaction to the computer; 133 clinicians, 23 percent of those who agreed to participate, took the time to type a comment. Comments were almost always favorable. "The computer is one of the greatest assets of Beth Israel Hospital," wrote one enthusiastic intern. "I just find it more convenient (and fun!) to look up the lab results I need using the computer terminal," typed a nurse from one of the medical units. "When I was an intern here, we didn't have the computer system like this. If we had, I estimate that I would have saved myself an hour a day at least," commented a medical resident. "A computer [terminal] should be installed in the dialysis unit," typed a staff nephrologist—and we had one installed as quickly as possible.

Democracy and the Computer Interview

At the time of the survey, it occurred to me that—Orwell's tyrannical Big Brother notwithstanding—the computer-based survey could actually be democratizing. One of the reasons for representational government is logistical: as a population grows, there comes a time when there are too many people to fit into a town hall. Lots of people can sit in front of interactive terminals, however, and computers are increasingly available—to people from all walks of life, both at work and at home. And the use of worldwide computing networks for interpersonal communication is flourishing. It seemed to me at the time that the computer could be used to empower people, offering them greater participation; with the computer, people could vote *on* issues rather than *for* representatives.

I would still argue that the computer-administered interview, used wisely and with care, is a valuable means of eliciting opinions about a wide variety of topics—in confidence and with anonymity if desired. And so it has been for users of the CCC system.

CYBERMEDICINE AND QUALITY OF CARE

The quality of medical care is, of course, our reason for being. It is also the most difficult process to measure. Difficult as this may be, however, those of us who work in the field of clinical computing, and those who market computing systems that purport to help in patient care, must face this issue head on and do our best to answer the question: Is the computer helping to improve the quality of medical care? Is the computer helping the patient in matters of health and illness?

Indirect Evidence

If it can be agreed that doctors for the most part engage in their diagnostic efforts with good reason and good will and with beneficial results for their patients, then the computing system that offers them the information they have requested, with more ease, speed, reliability, and accuracy than is otherwise possible, is improving the quality of care. The extensive, intensive voluntary use by clinicians at Beth Israel Deaconess and Brigham and Women's hospitals is convincing if indirect evidence that computing is making things better for doctors and patients.

Direct Evidence

Direct evidence is harder to come by. The efforts to date in our hospitals have been in studying the effect of advice, suggestions, alerts, and reminders offered to clinicians when they are using the computing systems. David Bates, Gilad Kuperman, Jonathan Teich, and their colleagues at Brigham and Women's Hospital have found that the time to act on important clinical events, such as critically abnormal laboratory results, is substantially reduced when your physician is alerted by the computer of the need to act. They have also found that physicians, who now routinely use their computing system to order laboratory tests and prescribe medications, are far less likely to make errors, including serious errors, with the tests they order and the medications they prescribe if they are apprised by the computer on the spot of the possibility of error. The investigators' findings indicate that their alerting system has reduced serious errors in medications at Brigham and Women's Hospital by *55 percent.*

At Beth Israel Deaconess Medical Center the alerts and reminders that are offered automatically to the appropriate doctors at the time they sign on to the CCC system have also proved helpful. Consider, for example, the situation discussed earlier where you are taking gentamicin for an infection and you have been found to have an abnormally high serum creatinine level, indicating that the gentamicin may be harming your kidneys as a toxic side effect. If an automatic alert about this situation leads your doctor to change the drug or reduce the dosage of gentamicin, the quality of medicine has been improved for you.

Under the direction of David Rind and Charles Safran, CCC investigators studied the effects of alerts and reminders on physicians who were confronted with such a situation. Doctors who received the alerts took substantially less time to change or discontinue kidney-related medications than did doctors who were not offered the alerts.

In a like manner, the time to act on clinical events such as the need for a flu vaccine or referral for an eye exam was substantially shorter when the doctor was reminded by the computing system of the need to act. Furthermore, the alerts and reminders have been well received by physicians as judged by their responses to a computer-conducted survey. Accordingly, we conclude that computer-delivered alerts and reminders beneficially affect physician behavior and thereby improve the quality of medical care.

Errors in Medicine

In the fall of 1999, the Institute of Medicine—one of the National Academies chartered by the U.S. Congress—issued a report titled *To Err Is Human* that presented startling data on the incidence of errors in medicine. The report concluded that "as many as 98,000 people die in any given year from medical errors that occur in hospitals." While the extent of the problem is debatable, most would agree that *iatrogenic conditions*—the occurrence of inadvertently induced, untoward events during the course of medical care—has received insufficient attention over the years and that preventable mistakes, in particular, should be at once addressed and redressed as soon as possible with intelligence and dispatch.

When it comes to mistakes made by physicians, there are two possible approaches from the behaviorist's perspective. One is to expose and criticize the perpetrator. The other, far better approach is to rein-force correct behavior—to make it as easy as possible for the doctor to practice good medicine. Most doctors want to do the best they can on behalf of patients, and anything that can make this easier will be a powerful reinforcing stimulus. Furthermore, existential considerations aside, punishment is a relatively ineffective means to bring about a desirable change in behavior of lasting value.

It has been suggested that we need to improve our methods of dis-closing medical errors—that better reporting will help thoughtful people, both at a federal and local level, evaluate important mistakes and develop measures to prevent future occurrence. While full dis-closure is an admirable goal, and good strategies are perhaps likely to accrue from further study, I would argue that we know enough already to greatly reduce important errors in medicine through the good use of cybermedicine. If the cybermedicine programs available to your doctor provide the results of diagnostic studies immediately upon request, with abnormal and critical values sufficiently high-lighted to avoid their being overlooked; if the programs offer unso-licited alerts and reminders about clinical events that need attention either immediately or in the near future; if the programs offer advice and consultation, when requested, about diagnosis and treatment; if the programs offer ready access to current, reliable medical litera-ture; if the programs offer access to information about the diagno-sis and treatment of patients from the past (with protection of confidentiality) for comparison with the diagnosis and treatment of patients in the present; if the programs assist with (or better, elimi-nate) administrative chores, thereby freeing more time for medical matters; and if the programs have educational value, your doctor is far less likely to make mistakes in the practice of medicine. No cyber-medicine system I know of achieves all these goals to the optimal extent, and there is much research to be done (keep those grants coming, if you please). But your doctor can have access to much of this cybermedicine in the near future, if the managerial, administra-tive, political, and territorial barriers can be overcome. But more of those shortly.

THE TEACHING POWER OF CYBERMEDICINE

In the tradition of John Dewey, who advocated "learning by doing," our cybermedicine systems promote learning in the context of caring for real patients rather than in the isolation of the classroom. At any time of day or night, a medical student or physician in training at Beth Israel Deaconess Medical Center or Brigham and Women's Hospital can look up information on the computer. Suppose that an intern caring for an elderly man at Beth Israel Deaconess is informed by the computer that his patient has low serum sodium and blood urea nitrogen concentrations and a chest X-ray film that shows enlarged lymph nodes at the base of one lung with fluid along the surface— findings suggestive of a lung cancer that is secreting a hormone normally secreted only by the pituitary gland. The intern can use the computer to get expert consultation on diagnosis and treatment (data from the laboratories and clinical departments are transferred to the consultation programs automatically), use ClinQuery to find information from other patients (with confidentiality protected) with these abnormalities, use PaperChase to search for related articles in the medical literature, and use e-mail to communicate with other clinicians in the hospital. Medical students and physicians in training use our cybermedicine system thousands of times each day, learning from the computer while helping in the practice of medicine.

COST OF CYBERMEDICINE

We have done our best to keep the costs of the cybermedicine systems as low as possible while providing computing that has the *primary purpose* of helping clinicians care for patients. During the developmental years in the 1980s, the total cost at Beth Israel Hospital was approximately 1.5 percent of the operating budget. At Brigham and Women's Hospital, where financial programs were also included, the cost was approximately 2 percent of the operating budget.

By comparison, our surveys indicate that hospitals tend to spend 2 percent to 6 percent of their yearly operating budget on computing. This computing is all too often limited to financial programs and patient registration, with perhaps a stand-alone laboratory system here or there, but with nothing much of use to the clinician.

EFFECT OF CYBERMEDICINE ON HOSPITAL FINANCES

In keeping with the budgetary wisdom of high-priced consultants that permeates clinical facilities these days, most computing in hospitals and clinics begins and ends with the financial department. In our experience, however, and what we know of the experience of others, financial computing is not well suited to the clinical needs of the doctor and patient. It is difficult if not impossible to direct the large mainframe computer in the billing department to the needs of the clinician.

It makes more sense to start with a cybermedical goal—helping the doctor help the patient. Not only is this what medicine is all about, but the finances of a clinical facility are better served when the financial computing is a *by-product* of the clinical system. The results of a diagnostic study, a red blood count, for example, represent more complex information than the amount to be charged for the study. It is easier for the computer to affix the charge to the study when the primary goal is to get the results to the doctor than to affix the study to the charge when the primary goal is to get the charge to the payer. In our experience, cybermedicine results in better financial accountability as well as better medicine.

At Beth Israel, the time required to collect unpaid bills (the amount of money not yet collected divided by the mean amount of the charges added per day) dropped from sixty-five days in 1977, when the registration component of the CCC system was first introduced, to thirty-nine days in 1982. Furthermore, as the number of patients being cared for and the number of diagnostic tests being performed has increased over the years, the number of employees in the admitting offices, the medical records department, and the clinical departments and laboratories has remained relatively stable in conjunction with the labor-saving power of the cybermedicine programs.

At Brigham and Women's Hospital, the time required to collect unpaid bills was reduced from a hundred days in 1983 to fifty-nine days in 1988. Outstanding debts in the ambulatory clinics were reduced by more than $6 million during a period when the cash collected from ambulatory patient revenues increased by 45 percent. Furthermore, the programs for clinicians have had a dramatically beneficial effect on hospital finances while improving the quality of medical care. The computer-based order-entry system developed by David Bates and his colleagues at Brigham and Women's is a striking example. Whereas the system costs the hospital about $2 million a year to maintain, it has saved the hospital approximately $5 million a year in accounts payable; and at the same time, the system has reduced a substantial number of important medical errors.

—〜〜—

Let us turn now to the clinician on-line with the Internet, PaperChase, and e-mail.

CHAPTER NINE

The Clinician On-Line

⁓

As it is for the patient, more and more medical information is available for the clinician by means of computer-based telecommunication—and, contrary to popular conception, physicians are far from being reluctant users. A recent survey by Nua Internet Surveys (http://www.nua.ie/surveys) indicated that 90 percent of physicians in the United States went on-line during the year 2000 and that 55 percent of physicians are daily Internet users.

Web sites available to the patient—the National Library of Medicine (http://www.nlm.nih.gov), the Centers for Disease Control and Prevention (http://www.cdc.gov), and Healthfinder (http://www.healthfinder.gov) from the Department of Health and Human Services, as three good examples—offer a wealth of information to the clinician as well. Multiple additional sites offer yet more information on a wide range of medical topics. Ironically, because of the unfortunate lack of good cybermedicine in so many of the hospitals and clinics in the United States, clinicians often have more access to medical information over the Internet than within the walls of their own facilities.

Most of the health-related material on the Internet is presented with limited interaction with the user. Much of what is available on-line is also available in pamphlets, textbooks, and other medical publications; to date, few medical journals are transmitted in their entirety. And of course the doctor (like any other user) must consider the source of the literature and be wary of misinformation. But in no way do I mean to demean the power of this resource for the clinician, which offers ready access to a vast amount of reading matter, much of it accurate and informative, available over the Internet at any time of day or night, seven days a week, fifty-two weeks a year.

THE NATIONAL INSTITUTES OF HEALTH

The Web site of the National Institutes of Health (http://www.nih.gov) offers Health Information, which provides information on health-related topics from "A" (beginning with abetalipoproteinemia, a genetic disorder characterized by an absence of important proteins in the blood) to "Z" (ending with zoonoses, infections that are shared between people and other animals). The Health Information section offers current wisdom on the management of a broad range of common important medical problems such as urinary incontinence, benign prostatic hyperplasia, early HIV infection, cancer pain, and low back pain. The Web site also includes Grants & Funding Opportunities, with information about how to apply for financial support for research; News & Events, with the results of clinical trials as soon as they are available; Scientific Resources, with descriptions of current research within the NIH; and Institutes, Centers & Offices, with descriptions of the organizational components of the NIH.

PAPERCHASE

How does information of use to the clinician and patient find its way to the Internet? My favorite example is PaperChase, a program whose purpose was to give people the ability to search the medical literature. I am not a disinterested observer. The inventor of PaperChase, Howard Bleich, has been my colleague in cybermedicine for over thirty years. But I consider PaperChase to be among the most important contributions to emerge from the field of cybermedicine.

In 1966, the National Library of Medicine established MEDLINE, an electronic database of references to articles published in the world's best medical journals. For each article referenced, a medical librarian enters into MEDLINE the title, the authors, the journal (together with the page numbers, volume, and year of publication), and the medical subject headings (MeSH terms), which are words assigned to help define the subject of an article. For example, "computers" is a MeSH term that would be assigned to an article about computers in medicine, even if the word "computer" did not appear in the title of the article. (The full text of articles is not part of MEDLINE, because of the great amount of electronic storage this would require.)

Each month, twenty-five thousand new references are indexed and abstracted. MEDLINE now has over nine million references to articles from over forty-three hundred journals. Bringing together as it does the world's medical articles that have been published in accredited journals, MEDLINE has been a powerful contribution from our federal government to the practice of medicine and to medical research.

As designed by the staff of the National Library of Medicine, MEDLINE was to be used by highly trained medical librarians who were experienced with the complex programming language (ELHILL) that permitted them to use the computer to search for articles; and until 1979, users of MEDLINE were required to consult with an experienced searcher, a librarian, who would serve as an intermediary and perform the desired searches. Such medical library resources were typically unavailable to patients and could be inconvenient, time-consuming, and expensive for clinicians and scientists—who would, after one or two tries, often revert to card catalogues and books such as the National Library's *Index Medicus* for help with their searches.

It was Howard's idea that people untrained as librarians and inexperienced with the use of computers could themselves search MEDLINE to good purpose. This was a radical idea for its time, and not all medical librarians accepted it. But to their credit, the librarians on the granting agency of the National Library, even those with reservations about the project, voted to give Howard and his coworkers financial support to develop his program.

An Observational Experiment

On August 1, 1979, Howard installed PaperChase on a computer terminal in the Beth Israel Hospital library. Patrons of the library, most of whom had never used such a terminal before, were then free to use it at any time of day or night. No instructions were provided, no users' manual was written, no announcements were made, and no publicity was given. On the screen was a message that read: "PaperChase: a computer program to help you search the medical literature. To start the program, press the ENTER key." The program itself was designed to be self-instructional and to offer advice and suggestions on how best to proceed.

Between 4 P.M. and midnight, 12 people signed on and performed searches; the next day, 39 people signed on and performed 75 searches. During the first year, 1,229 people performed 10,678 searches—more computerized searches of the MEDLINE database than were performed at any other institution in the country. During the third year, 2,202 people performed 16,803 searches. House officers were among the heaviest users.

Over the years, as the number of users grew, PaperChase was installed in the other Harvard teaching hospitals, and later in private offices and institutions throughout the United States and abroad. In the late 1980s, PaperChase was put on the Internet, and it now has its own Web site. On a typical weekday, there are now about 3,000 searches with PaperChase. Initially used primarily by clinicians and scientists, PaperChase is used increasingly by patients as well. Lawyers, administrators, and financial people are also among the growing ranks of those who seek access to the medical literature.

Since the inception of PaperChase, a number of commercially available products to search the medical literature have appeared on the market, and are available for use on the Internet as well as on stand-alone personal computers. And the National Library of Medicine now offers Grateful Med and Pub Med, its own general-purpose programs for access to MEDLINE.

E-MAIL

E-mail on the Internet is heavily used these days by clinicians as well as patients. There are newsgroups and mailing lists primarily for clinicians in virtually every specialty, and numerous newsgroups and mailing lists are shared by clinicians and patients in the spirit of partnership, collegiality, and self-help.

Increasingly, also, physicians are proffering medical advice to people over the Internet. This raises interesting issues concerning malpractice liability. Among the doctors I know who are providing this service on an informal basis with no fees involved, there is a consensus that this is a humanitarian service rather than a medical legal transaction. There have been no lawsuits to date that I know of. Would that this will remain the case.

With our own homegrown e-mail systems in use at Beth Israel Deaconess and Brigham and Women's hospitals, we have done observational studies that have given us some insights into the dynamics of this powerful new form of communication.

E-Mail in Two Teaching Hospitals

As mentioned in Chapter Seven, CCC e-mail was developed in the late 1970s as part of our cybermedicine system and was implemented first at Beth Israel Hospital and then at Brigham and Women's. The idea was that e-mail would help the people in the admitting and medical records departments communicate with each other and with those of us in cybermedicine who were working with them to develop and maintain their systems. None of us, however, realized the extent to which e-mail would revolutionize communication. As more and more programs were added to the CCC system, as more and more terminals were available, and as more and more people were signing on to use the programs in their day-to-day activities throughout the hospital and ambulatory clinics, the number of users of e-mail and the extent of their use grew dramatically. Electronic mail was being pulled by those who wanted to use it; it was not being pushed by those who designed it, who were content to observe in amazement.

With our earliest version of e-mail, each user with a password could write and read messages to other password holders. Shortly thereafter, at the request of the users, we added the ability to send messages to individually compiled lists of people, to lists of members of one or more departments, or when deemed necessary, to all holders of passwords who were affiliated with the hospital. For example, an instructor in psychiatry could establish a list of medical students and then use this option to forward advice to the group or invite them to a teaching session; each student, in turn, could acknowledge receipt of the advice, perhaps ask some questions, or indicate plans to attend. A chief resident in medicine could notify all residents that an instructive, unscheduled conference was about to occur, and a technologist in the blood bank could notify all who signed on that there was an urgent need for a particular type of blood.

Soon additional features were added. At the time of signing on, each user was informed about new mail and offered the opportunity to read it then or later. Users could send mail immediately or post it for future delivery. They could store mail that had been read in folders of their choice for future use; they could view messages previously sent, and reread their old mail; and they could edit messages received and then forward them to others.

We also incorporated two options that have been very helpful in our experience but are still not commonly part of other e-mail systems. Inquire If Message Read enables you to determine whether your message has been received. This is particularly helpful if you have not yet received a reply to a message of importance. Retract Mail enables you to cancel a message if it has not yet been read and you have second thoughts about sending it or would like to make changes. With the retract option you can experience the psychological benefit of a verbal catharsis—after sending a note in anger, for example—without suffering the diplomatic consequences. Once the message has been read, of course, the proverbial die is cast. (The neurologist in me is looking for a way to retrieve the message *after* it has been read, but I have been unsuccessful to date.)

In some cases the computer itself now generates messages. When a patient is readmitted or seen in the emergency room, a message to that effect automatically goes to all physicians on whose Personal Patient List the patient's name appears. Physicians have told us that they very much appreciate this feature; it alerts them when one of their patients returns to the hospital, even if under the care of another physician, and it eliminates the need for them to telephone the emergency room repeatedly to find out whether an expected patient has arrived.

Assessing Use

As with our other cybermedicine programs, we like to evaluate the e-mail system by how often it is used by voluntary users—those whose jobs do not require using it. And use has been extensive. During the week of February 23 to 29, 1992, a total of 2,354 clinicians at Beth Israel Hospital—1,022 nurses, 523 health assistants, 305 house officers, 352 staff physicians, 103 clinical fellows, and 49 medical students—sent in the range of 20,000 pieces of e-mail. By 1996, four years later, they were sending over 30,000 messages a week. Those who were most directly involved in patient care were the heaviest users. And at Brigham and Women's Hospital, use has been equally extensive.

During a computer-conducted survey at Beth Israel in 1992, 90 percent of those surveyed indicated that the e-mail system "made life easier" for them and 61 percent felt that e-mail had actually had a "human-izing influence" on their lives. Furthermore, many favorable comments about e-mail have come our way *by* e-mail. "This has been a very help-ful service and has added to our ability to provide good care, [to] communicate . . . and has been a real time saver as well," wrote a staff physician in obstetrics and gynecology at Brigham and Women's Hospital.

Although most of the messages sent and received are related to patient care or other issues that pertain to work within a clinical facil-ity, personal messages are common as well, and this I would argue is all to the good. Personnel in hospitals and clinics work under emo-tionally stressful conditions, and e-mail, by facilitating interpersonal communication, can serve to relieve debilitating pressure and engen-der feelings of well-being. At both hospitals, a rapidly growing num-ber of people with specialized interests have developed e-mail lists for intercommunication. In these institutions, where the primary goal is the care of others, e-mail groups serve the purpose of self-care as well—an electronic form of group therapy, much like the mailing lists that have evolved on the Internet. Designed originally for intramural use, our homegrown e-mail system, the cybermedicine lifeline within the walls of our hospitals, is now used as well for communication with the outside world by electronic connection with the Internet.

A Special Niche for E-Mail

In the clinical situation, when you must reach someone in a hurry—when there is a medical emergency, for example, and you need to get in touch with a doctor immediately—the best form of telecommuni-cation is the electronic "page," the beeper, or the portable cellular phone. When it is imperative that you talk with a person at the time of contact, there is still no substitute for the telephone. On the other hand, the telephone has its limitations. The person you are calling may be away from the phone, and you must then leave a message or take the time to call again. In turn, you may be away from the phone when the return call comes in, and you may continue in this mode, back and forth in a time-consuming process known as telephone tag. Further-more, your call may arrive at an inopportune time, when the person you are calling is available but otherwise occupied, thus forcing a choice between inconvenience at the moment or telephone tag in the future. And of course you can't edit what you have said on the phone. You can apologize and restate, but you can't retract.

When delays in conversation are acceptable, when you can wait a while between a message sent and a message received, e-mail fills what was heretofore a void in communication. With e-mail, you can read and write messages at your own convenience and with assurance of delivery. You can send a message at any time of day or night without worrying about interrupting the recipient, who in turn will read your message at a time of convenience, day or night. As many of the users of the CCC mail system have pointed out, telephone tag for them is a thing of the past.

With CCC e-mail you can take your time when composing, editing, and revising a message—and as I have mentioned earlier, if the message has been sent but not read, you can retract it and keep the repercussions of what you have said to a minimum. Furthermore, stored messages, both sent and received, can be kept as a permanent record of past conversations.

With e-mail, group discussions are easy to initiate. You can readily bring others into your conversation by amending, annotating, and forwarding messages without having to coordinate your schedules. People in groups can participate at their convenience. And e-mail can serve to promote common courtesy. In our experience, "Thank you" and "You're welcome" are easily (and therefore often) transmitted—and much appreciated.

Well-meaning voices of concern are sometimes raised about e-mail. Will it depersonalize conversation? Will it dehumanize interpersonal relationships? Will people stop talking to each other? It is helpful to remember, therefore, that e-mail is an adjunct to face-to-face communication, not a replacement. It permits conversation when face-to-face communication is impossible, and when the telephone is impractical. Carefully written e-mail messages can improve working conditions and interpersonal relationships as well.

Potential Problems with E-Mail

Not all is right with e-mail, of course. First of all, it takes at least two people to use it. If you send a message to someone who rarely reads e-mail, if your message falls on blind eyes, so to speak, the advantages are lost. However, where thousands of people are using the computer each day for a wide variety of purposes and where e-mail is one of many available options, as it is with the cybermedicine systems at our two hospitals, e-mail becomes part of the routine and messages are read and written with high volume and consistent regularity. In our experience, it is the rare user who doesn't turn repeatedly to e-mail, day in and day out.

The second issue is unsolicited (read junk) e-mail. You may get more electronic messages than you care to read. Cognitive overload is of real concern to us these days as we attempt to sift and winnow the information that confronts us. (It has been estimated that there is more information available to the reader of one issue of the *New York Sunday Times* than was available to any literate person throughout the entire eighteenth century.) It is imperative, therefore, that users of any e-mail system be able to dissociate themselves from mailing lists that yield unwanted material. Users should be able to search on-line for information they want and need, from the bulletin board to the interactive encyclopedia, but at the same time, they should be protected from masses of unsolicited materials that serve only to clutter the mind.

Third, there is the emotive aspect of e-mail. Just as we noticed years ago that people are sometimes more comfortable with a computer than they are with a doctor while answering questions of a potentially embarrassing nature, there is a tendency for some people to emote more freely by e-mail than they would in person. Sometimes the most mild-mannered, gentle person will let go at the computer with a tirade that would never occur face to face, like the humble pedestrian who becomes a hostile antagonist behind the wheel of a car. And sometimes people will send messages that are just plain ill-advised, messages that may come back to haunt them.

Fourth, there is the issue of the attractive nuisance. Will people waste their time with e-mail? Will teleconverse supplant more useful human endeavors? Will it be used for mischief? In this regard, I would submit that e-mail is a neutral medium, which can be misused if people set out to do so. But rather than regulating its use—protecting people from themselves, as it were—I hope we can devote our energies to encouraging and reinforcing the gainful uses of this powerful new means of communication.

Finally, in spite of best intentions, there can be no certain protection of the confidentiality of any e-mail message in any system, although with our CCC cybermedicine system we have taken all the protective measures we could envision.

Having touched on the issue of confidentiality, I think it's time to pursue this essential issue further. How can we best protect privacy? How can we protect confidential clinical information once it has been placed in a computer?

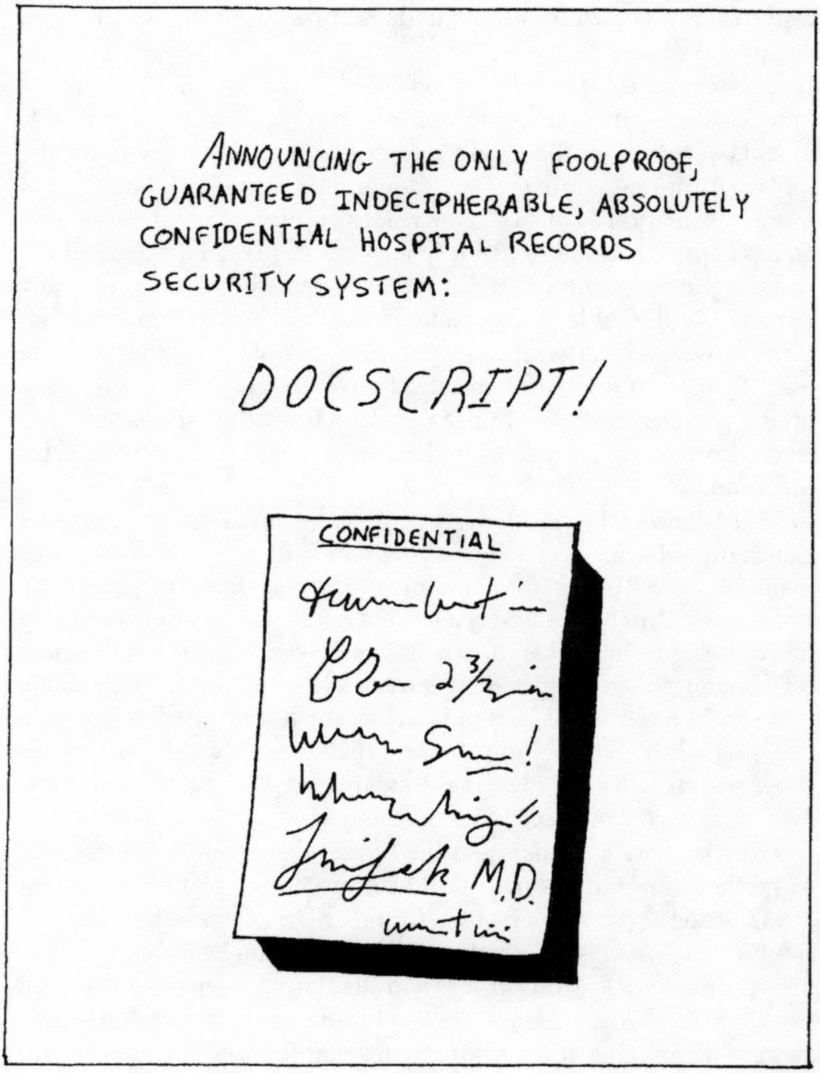
ANNOUNCING THE ONLY FOOLPROOF, GUARANTEED INDECIPHERABLE, ABSOLUTELY CONFIDENTIAL HOSPITAL RECORDS SECURITY SYSTEM:
DOCSCRIPT!
CONFIDENTIAL
M.D.

Confidentiality

J oe Louis once quipped about a forthcoming opponent, "He can run but he can't hide." Today the world is even more of a metaphorical ring, a place where we can run but we can't hide. Big Brother hovers over us, ready to descend at any time.

In days gone by, a man who was out of favor in his hometown could pick up stakes and move to another community. There he could start anew, unencumbered by past transgressions or other best-forgotten aspects of his personal history; he could achieve geographic anonymity, if you will. When a person went west to the New World in the eighteenth century, or west to the Pacific in the nineteenth century, this was as much to escape the past as to find the future. Part of the American dream in those days was the chance to start fresh. Even the outlaw on the loose could find safe haven in a Hole in the Wall or a Teneke Springs. Now our pasts are with us for life, ready to be made public by interested parties if we don't take action to stop them. By "them" I mean those who would chip away at our Bill of Rights or stand by as others chip away, who would condone the use of technology, be it the telephone tap or the computer data bank, to intrude on our private lives, including our medical records.

Now if people want to find you and have the resources to do so, they can not only find you but find out all about you. Virtually anyone can get access to your social security number. (In Massachusetts, it's the number on your driver's license unless you take action to object.) On-line services on the Internet offer access to your demographic information (an on-line "White Pages" shows your house on a map). Banks, credit companies, testing companies, and the Internal Revenue Service obtain enough information as part of routine operations to compile financial, educational, and occupational biographies of us all. And this is not to mention how much information a reporter, a detective, or an FBI agent can obtain.

There is, of course, a gray zone between justified intrusion on behalf of the law and unjustified intrusion by a snoop or ideologue. This is part of the age-old conflict between the interests of society and the rights of the individual. But to paraphrase Samuel Johnson, just because you can't tell the difference between dusk and dawn doesn't mean you can't tell the difference between night and day. We know a snoop when we see one.

Those of us who believe strongly in the right to privacy must do our best to guard against unwarranted intrusion and fight back when it occurs. At the least we should speak out against the snoops and let *them* be the objects of public scrutiny.

THE MEDICAL RECORD

Just as no one can guarantee our privacy in other aspects of life, no one can guarantee the privacy of our medical records, whether they are on paper or in a computer. Once medical information is recorded in any form, it is subject to being divulged, despite the best intentions of the clinicians involved. The clinical transaction is no longer a simple relationship between patient and doctor. Even with a routine checkup, the receptionist knows the appointment has been made, the laboratory technologist knows the results of the blood test, the X-ray technologist knows how the film has been interpreted, and the pharmacist knows which medications have been prescribed. These people, as well as the doctor, may all be committed to the protection of privacy, but leaks can and do occur.

In the past, it seemed as though everyone *but* the patient had access to the medical record; the clinician, the hospital administrator, the insurance company, the lawyer, or the government could lay claim to it more easily than the patient could. This situation is changing today. More and more patients have access to their medical records, some-times even with editing privileges—if not with the right to delete, at least with the right to correct and append.

Some people don't mind if their medical records are available to others. Individuals differ widely when it comes to the need for privacy. For one person, pregnancy may be a joyous event happily related to others; for another it is something to hide. And many patients suffer from the stigma associated with some illnesses and most emotional problems. It would of course be better if there was no stigma associated with illness. Perhaps we can see to it that illnesses no longer need to be kept secret. Perhaps the Thomas Eagletons of the future can seek help for depression and still run for vice president. I hope this will come to pass.

Patients do have some control over the information that goes *into* their medical records—you don't have to tell your doctor everything, and you can refuse to undergo diagnostic study. Still, to get help from a doctor or a policy from a life insurance company you may have to divulge information that you would prefer to keep private.

The conflict between the rights of the individual and the interests of the group is especially apparent in the area of infectious diseases and behavioral disorders, in which one person's problem can adversely affect another. When one sailor with smallpox was put ashore on the east coast of the Queen Charlotte Islands in 1860, the population in Haida villages there was almost destroyed within a period of several years. In such cases, as with other social conflicts, we must turn to the law for guidance, though only with extreme caution. When, for exam-ple, are public disclosure and quarantine justified in the effort to safe-guard society? Still, most of us would agree that when it comes to most decisions about divulging information to people who are not involved in patient care, the patient should be in charge.

In the best of circumstances all medical information should be kept confidential, known only to those with good reasons to know. But there is a need for compromise here. There is a direct relationship between the usefulness of a medical record in the practice of medi-cine and its potential for unwarranted disclosure. The easier it is to retrieve the information in the record, the less secure it is from breaches of privacy. To put this another way, the more easily an autho-rized clinician can make good use of a patient's record, the more eas-ily an unauthorized person can make bad use of it. With this fine line, too little protection of confidentiality will compromise your privacy as a patient, but too much will compromise the quality of your care.

The Paper Record

The traditional paper chart, when at its best in protecting confidentiality, is at its worst as a useful medical record. The best defense against unauthorized intrusion into the paper chart is the illegibility of the doctors' handwriting; I have trouble reading my own handwriting, not to mention that of my colleagues, and I am not alone in this. Coupled with illegibility is the traditional disorganization of the paper chart. Since there is usually no index or table of contents, whatever information *can* be read is still difficult to retrieve and use.

On the other hand, if the paper chart is legible and well organized, as it is in a few exceptional hospitals and clinics, it is also more vulnerable to breach of privacy. Virtually anyone with a white coat, a name tag, and an imposing facial expression can walk into a nursing station, pull a patient's chart from the rack, and read it without being questioned—as a *Boston Globe* reporter did some years ago in a local hospital. Even Nurse Ratched would hesitate to confront such an intruder. Doctors don't like to be questioned, and anyone with a white coat and a name tag might be a doctor.

The Record in the Computer

The ultimate confidential computer would be a computer with no output. Many doctors and nurses have seen computers in medicine that behave as if they had no output. These machines are sometimes advertised as if this lack of output were an advantage—"complex encryption prevents access by unauthorized users." If you can crack the "complex encryption," you find that it has been protecting very little of any use—a situation reminiscent of Dick Gregory's experience during the civil rights years: he waited and waited at the whites-only lunch counter, and when at long last the staff acknowledged him, they didn't have anything he wanted. At the other end of the spectrum would be the computer with unlimited output, one that yielded anyone's medical record to anyone who requested it, which of course would be at least as unacceptable.

In any clinical facility that houses patients' medical records, three groups of people, in addition to the patient or a designated surrogate, may want access to a patient's record:

- Those with no legitimate reason to see any part of any patient's record. This group includes nonclinical personnel, visitors, and intruders.

- Those whose jobs entail using a limited portion of the patient's record. This group includes the receptionist who makes the patient's appointment, the laboratory technologist who needs the blood count but not the results of the gonorrhea culture, and the billing person who needs to know the charge for an HIV test but not the results. (The fact that this person knows that a patient has even had an HIV test is of course a privacy issue in its own right.)

- Those who need access to the entire records of the patients under their care but should not see the records of other patients.

PROTECTING CONFIDENTIALITY WITHIN THE HOSPITAL AND CLINIC

When the medical record is in the computer, those responsible for the computing system must keep intrusion to a minimum while helping appropriate, authorized clinicians find the information they need. With our CCC cybermedicine systems at Beth Israel Deaconess Medical Center and Brigham and Women's Hospital, we have done our best both to protect patient confidentiality and to enhance the quality of patient care.

Preventing Access by Intruders

Each authorized user of the computers at the two hospitals and their related clinics and private offices gains access to the cybermedicine system by means of a unique, computer-assigned, confidential password. Only a few people in supervisory positions can instruct the computer to issue a password. The computer does this because we have learned that people who choose their own passwords tend to use their initials or another sequence that is easy for them to remember, but also easy for someone else to guess. The computer constructs a password out of consonants (no vowels) to make it intentionally difficult to memorize, in case it is deliberately or inadvertently observed. Typically the user invents a mnemonic to help with recall. A user can ask the computer for a new password at any time, and will routinely receive a new password every six months.

All users are advised that a password is equivalent to a personal signature, and that under no circumstances should it be shared with anyone. The extensive use of e-mail in the hospitals and clinics, for personal as well as job-related purposes, provides another incentive to keep our passwords to ourselves; when passwords are shared, the wrong people can read our e-mail.

The computers at the two hospitals maintain a dictionary of passwords and the names of their owners. If an unauthorized person repeatedly tries to use an illegal password, the terminal beeps the Morse code for "SOS" eighteen times and stops responding to its keyboard. It stays unusable until someone at the computer center releases the software lock. With the use of passwords, we are putting a higher priority on confidentiality than on patient care; the need to enter a password slows the clinician's access to needed information.

Restricting Access According to Need

Each password permits access only to programs appropriate for its owner, and then only from terminals appropriate for those programs. For example, a password assigned to a laboratory technologist permits access only to programs in that laboratory, and then only from terminals located there; a password assigned to a hematology technologist does not permit access to results from the microbiology laboratory.

Some passwords can be used only for looking at data, some can be used to enter and edit data, and some can be used to issue new passwords. After a user has completed a transaction such as scheduling an appointment, assigning a room, or correcting a patient's identifying information in the registry, the password must be entered as a personal signature—another incentive not to share it. The computer then records the date, the time, the name of the person who performed the transaction, the program used, and the location of the terminal.

Access by Authorized Clinicians

Only the doctors, nurses, and other clinicians who are participating directly in a patient's care, or those who are authorized to do clinical research with the informed consent of the patient, have a legitimate reason to gain access to a patient's computer-based medical record. It might seem reasonable, therefore, to restrict each clinician's access to patients who are known to be under his or her care. On the other hand, in an urgent situation, any clinician in the hospital might need to care for any patient. A doctor might be called away suddenly or otherwise unavailable, or an emergency might arise that would require all available clinical help.

Accordingly, we decided that the password of each authorized clinician would permit access to the clinical data of all patients in the hospital registry. In so doing, we have given a higher priority to the quality of a patient's care than to the protection of the patient's privacy. Any staff doctor could look up information in the medical record of a colleague or a celebrity without a legitimate reason to do so.

However, we have taken steps to make such intrusion unlikely. On receiving their first password, clinicians all sign a computer-generated document promising not to look at clinical information unnecessarily. In addition, whenever a clinician looks up a patient's data, the transaction is recorded in the computer and is, on request, made available to the patient or the patient's physician. Furthermore, if the patient is thought to be in need of special protection—is a hospital employee, a family member of a hospital employee, or a celebrity—the computer displays a reminder that is applicable to all patients:

> To protect each patient's confidentiality, only those who are responsible for a patient's care should use this option. We record the identity of each user of Patient Lookup and will give this information to the patient or the patient's physician upon request.

In addition, from time to time the computer selects a patient at random and transmits the same message. With this admonition, a potential unwarranted intrusion, particularly if it is innocent, can be averted.

All staff members of Beth Israel Deaconess and Brigham and Women's hospitals are themselves potential patients in the hospitals and are therefore included in the common registry of patients in the computing systems. It can be argued that these people need special protection from unwarranted intrusion by fellow hospital workers. Accordingly, we have implemented as a utility in the computing systems an option labeled View Lookups Of Your Own File. This option, which is used several hundred times each week, enables everyone on the staff to determine who has obtained access to their own clinical records in the computer.

In the ambulatory setting at Beth Israel Deaconess, Jonathan Wald and his coworkers in the CCC added a feature—of particular appeal to those in psychiatry and psychology—whereby the author of an electronic note can designate it as "monitored." The author of a monitored note will receive an automatic message providing the name of each person who reads it, the date and time of the viewing, and the reason the person gives for looking at the note.

Loopholes Beyond Our Control

Our approach to confidentiality is based on physical protection—most computer terminals are located in supervised areas—and on the use of individual passwords. But we have also relied on personal accountability and trust, and this has proved to be justified. Known transgressions have been rare. Illegibility notwithstanding, we believe that computerized medical records can be better protected than paper charts. We are certain that they can be more helpful to clinicians.

Of more concern to me than the protection of confidentiality within the walls of a hospital is the protection of confidentiality once clinical information leaves the hospital. The Internet offers a powerful means of transmitting clinical information from doctor to doctor and from institution to institution for good medical reasons. Yet once confidential information is on the Internet, it becomes particularly vulnerable to unauthorized and unwarranted intrusion. Several efforts are currently under way to develop means to protect the confidentiality of medical records once they are transmitted over the Internet. In one of these, David Rind and his colleagues in the Boston Electronic Medical Record Collaborative have developed a protocol that would make it possible to permit access only to authorized clinicians with good reasons to know.

Of more concern to me still is the transmission of clinical information to nonclinical parties. For purposes of reimbursement, hospitals and clinics are now required to send confidential clinical information linked to charges out to a broad array of third-party payers—strangers, if you will, who are beyond the control of the hospital, doctor, or patient. Are they to be trusted?

IN THE HANDS OF STRANGERS

Before the Second World War, the fee-for-service system was the predominant means of payment for medical care in this country. The doctor billed and the patient paid, often on the spot. Most doctors developed their own fee systems, which depended on the patient's ability to pay. Payment was not always monetary. Commodities that the patient could afford—the proverbial bag of potatoes, for example—were sometimes accepted in lieu of cash. If a patient couldn't pay at all, the doctor would write off the bill, a form of socialized medicine, one on one. (A practice called "professional courtesy" meant that doctors would not bill or pay each other.) Only people who were directly involved in a patient's care—the doctor, the nurse, perhaps the office receptionist, and when needed, the local pharmacist—were privy to the patient's diagnosis and treatment. Confidentiality was based on a clinical ethic, a pact between the doctor and patient.

When a patient needed hospitalization, hospitals billed on a fee-for-service basis. Housing within the hospital was a function of a patient's payment status: *private,* a room to oneself for well-to-do patients; *semi-private,* a room shared with a few others, for middle-income patients; and *charity,* a large open ward for patients who could not pay. The private hospital catered to the affluent. The charity hospital, typically large and city-supported, was the medical repository for the poor.

In teaching hospitals, whether private or public, charity patients were part of the educational process; medical students, interns, and residents were their primary physicians. Charity patients were used for instructional purposes in surgery and obstetrics as well as internal medicine, in return for free medical care. This was sometimes to the patient's advantage. What the medical student lacked in experience could be compensated for, at least in part, by careful devotion to the task. Furthermore, in good teaching hospitals, the interns supervised the students, the residents supervised the interns, and an experienced staff physician supervised the group and was available to provide direct patient care when needed. What was lost in comfort—multiple examinations day and night by multiple doctors in training—could be gained in comprehensiveness; with all the redundancy, it was unlikely that something important would be overlooked.

The large open charity wards were short on personal privacy. The curtains around the beds were flimsy, and confidential conversations were overheard by patients in adjacent beds and by their visitors. (Unfortunately loose talk among clinicians in corridors, stairways, and elevators is still a common source of breach of confidentiality.) On the other hand, there was a clear distinction between those who had legitimate reasons to look at a patient's chart and those who did not—that is, those who were responsible for a patient's care and those who were not. For the most part, confidential information for all hospitalized patients was kept within the walls of the hospital. Patients trusted the hospital to protect their privacy. Breaches of confidentiality, when they occurred, occurred inside the hospital.

But this is no longer the case. Since the advent of medical insurance, the walls of a hospital are no longer a protective barrier against loss of privacy. A third party has arrived on the scene, a party of strangers from outside the clinical sanctum. And *they* insist on having access to patients' medical records.

You Bet Your Health

Buying an insurance policy is a form of gambling. When you buy life insurance, the insurance company is betting you won't die within the term of the policy, but you are betting you will. When you buy automobile insurance, the insurance company is betting you won't have an accident, but you are betting you will. And when you buy medical insurance, the insurance company is betting you won't get sick, but you are betting you will. The game begins when you pay the premium (ante up) to the insurance company (the house); if you default on your premiums, the company keeps your money and you lose your policy. It is understood that the house usually wins; otherwise the game could not go on.

This is unusual gambling, to be sure; the incentives are perverse. When you're playing poker, you do everything you can to win (honestly, of course). When you're gambling on your health or life, by contrast, you don't try to win. But if you do win, you expect to get paid. As in other forms of gambling, cheating can occur and sometimes does. Insurance companies may delay or disallow payments for legitimate claims, and insured people need protection against this. On the other hand, insured people may make fraudulent claims, and insurance companies want protection against that. They want proof of what they are paying for.

With the evolution of medical insurance, clinicians and hospitals have found themselves constrained to give out confidential information from patients' medical records. The people who pay the bill are now the third party in the practice of medicine.

The Third Party

In the early days of medical insurance, during the 1940s and 1950s, the concept of a third-party payer was controversial, particularly within the medical profession. The concerns were not so much about privacy as about finance. The American Medical Association, as a union dutifully representing its physician members, was concerned that third-party payers would impose restrictions on fees. Group insurance programs such as the Kaiser Permanente Plan in California and the Health Insurance Plan in New York came under heavy criticism from the AMA, even to the point of organized boycotts.

With time, however, which brought rapidly rising medical costs and an increased demand for insurance coverage, medical insurance plans became more and more available both for individuals and for groups. And the number of private plans grew at a seemingly exponential rate. What were once a few tax-exempt programs, such as Blue Cross and Blue Shield, have now become a vast array of nonprofit and for-profit corporations. Even the federal government, despite opposition from the AMA and other forces of economic conservatism, became accepted as a principal player with the inception of Medicare in 1965. Universal coverage is now in demand, and third-party payers are more than ready to market their wares.

The new kid on the block, and in some instances already the bully, is the managed care company. Some for-profit and some tax-exempt, managed care companies now wield great power over health care delivery. Marketing its medical payment plan primarily to the employer who provides coverage for its employees, the managed care company can determine which clinicians are participants and what services are reimbursable. The managed care company wants to know what it's paying for. But further, by controlling the purse strings it is also managing the patient's care, at least indirectly. This is particularly evident in behavioral health where the treatment prescribed, even to the number of therapy sessions allowed, is dictated by the third-party payer.

All third-party payers have financial computers to help them out. In fact, their rapid growth has been to a large extent because of their computing facilities. Some insurance agencies and managed care companies market more than one plan. Massachusetts now has about three hundred medical coverage plans. Insurance buildings are going up at a rate rivaled only by banks. Hospitals and clinics are competing to provide services for the plans. Whatever else it may be, and by whatever name, medical insurance is big business in a sellers' market.

Managed care plans tend to reverse the financial incentives in the practice of medicine. In the days of fee-for-service payment, the more time spent, the more procedures done, and the longer the stay in the hospital, the higher the fee. As a result, too much was sometimes done and inefficiency was not discouraged. With managed care, the less time spent, the fewer procedures done, and the shorter the stay in the hospital, the higher the profits (or nonprofit profits) for the payer. In hospitals and clinics with managed care plans, the financial incentive is to stick to the practice plans prescribed by the managed care company; cost overruns are absorbed by the hospital.

Universal Coverage

Despite the problems inherent in all medical payment plans, there is general agreement these days that the United States and its people would be far better off if we could all have medical coverage, regardless of our finances. We should all be protected from financial ruin if a medical catastrophe strikes us or a family member. Those who would otherwise be unable to pay for their medical care should no longer be dependent on the beneficence of their doctors and hospital facilities.

Third-party payers foster consistency in payment among patients, regardless of their personal financial situation, so that the distinction now is between insured and uninsured patients rather than rich and poor. Large open wards, even in charity hospitals, have for the most part disappeared, a relic of the past. Insured patients can choose their own doctor (within the limits of their plan) and can insist that the role of "teaching patient" be shared by all patients alike.

Whether there should be many insurance houses, such as we have in the United States, or one house—the government—and whether we should ante up directly through premiums, or indirectly through our employers or government, are hotly contested issues. But there is general agreement that those who have medical coverage are better off than those who don't, and that we must find a way to cover everyone for major medical expenses. (As a means of keeping the costs down, a strong argument can be made for some direct fee-for-service payments for those who can afford it.)

But we must also confront the issue of privacy. The third-party payer in medical care, in whatever form it may take—government or private, for profit or not for profit—represents a breach in the traditional pact of confidentiality between doctor and patient.

Beyond the Clinical Sanctum

Most medical facilities ask each of their patients to sign a release form giving them permission to send a patient's medical information to whatever agency will be paying the bill. All third-party payers require the patient's name and other personally identifying information, which they use to verify that there was in fact a clinical transaction. In addition, the payer insists on knowing the medical diagnosis (at the very least), which is typically transmitted in the form of an ICD-9 code (*International Classification of Diseases,* ninth revision).

Moreover, the information sent to the payer usually goes well beyond the medical diagnosis. Diagnostic and surgical procedures, laboratory tests performed, and medications prescribed are often included. The results of diagnostic studies are not usually provided, but the mere fact that a test was done—for AIDS, for example—can be highly revealing. The same is true with medications: if a man is taking AZT (zidovudine), it is not difficult to conclude that he has AIDS. Sometimes payers will go so far as to require the details of a patient's diagnosis and treatment. For example, a managed care plan may insist on a detailed psychiatric history from the clinician before covering the costs of psychotherapy.

Role of the Computer

In hospitals and practices that rely on traditional paper records, a manual process is used to send information to third-party payers—a process that is arduous and often inaccurate. In medical facilities that use computing in routine patient care, such as Beth Israel Deaconess and Brigham and Women's hospitals, the information is already available in electronic form. There is an irony here. Just as computer technology can make it easier to protect the privacy of patients within the walls of a hospital, so the technology makes it easier to breach their privacy outside these walls.

Trusting Strangers

The stated purpose of placing confidential medical information in the hands of third-party payers is to enable them to verify the legitimacy of financial claims. Little is known, however, about how the paying agencies protect the confidentiality of clinical information. Who within *and without* their walls has access to private information once it is in their computers? Do they use passwords? What are their procedures for issuing passwords? Do they keep track of use? How do they control against errors? How do they ensure accuracy?

I telephoned a number of insurance agencies in Massachusetts but have been unable to get answers to these questions. The usual response is, "We conform to the laws of the state of Massachusetts." When I ask "What laws?" they refer me to the state government. When I call the state government, I am referred back to the insurance agency.

We are faced with a conflict between two legitimate interests—the insurance agency's interest in protection against fraud and the patient's interest in privacy. So far the scales are tipped in favor of the insurance agencies.

From One Stranger to Another

Protection against fraud is understandable. But when confidential information is passed from one agency to another, without the explicit permission of the insured, a trust is broken. When a company that markets both medical insurance and life insurance disallows a life insurance policy on the basis of the information in the applicant's medical insurance record, the patient has reason to object. And when an insurance company disallows a life insurance policy on the basis of information obtained from *another* insurance company, the person has even more reason to object. Both these situations occur. It turns out that third-party payers routinely send confidential information in their computers to those of yet another agency.

The Medical Information Bureau is a tax-exempt corporation that stores medical information from approximately seven hundred member insurance agencies. Member agencies can query the Medical Information Bureau for information about their clients. In describing the bureau, P. S. Entmacher wrote that "safeguards are taken to assure confidentiality, and there is no linkage with other computer banks," but details on these safeguards are not provided. The medical information housed in the bureau is outside the control of the patient.

The Medical Information Bureau maintains a very low profile. Few people other than the member agencies even know of its existence. Few people, and I am not one of them, know how the bureau's information is used. Is it used to compile mailing lists? For marketing? For mischief? What are the safeguards for ensuring confidentiality? What are the safeguards for ensuring accuracy? We, the insured, are in the dark. Our privacy is beyond our control.

A Prescription for Privacy

It is time to achieve a better balance between the interests of the third-party payer and the interests of the patient. A legislative approach comes first to mind. Should we not turn to the government, state or federal, to pass laws that protect our confidentiality, laws that impose restrictions on what can be done with clinical information once it is in the hands of strangers? Indeed, some laws have already been passed, and others are on the way. But wait. Thomas Jefferson once observed that all too often when one law is introduced to solve one problem, two problems are created in its place. Who would enforce the laws? Would the laws spawn yet another government agency? Would we end up with a FCCMI, a Federal Commission on Confidential Medical Information—publicly funded, of course? Would its employees themselves need access to the confidential information? How else could they make certain that the insurance agencies were obeying the law?

I have another solution. Let's stop the problem at its source. *Let's stop sending confidential information to third-party payers, government or private.* We can develop a classification system that documents each clinical transaction, based on levels of severity of illness, but is free of clinical content. This would protect the third-party payer, within reason, as well as the privacy of the patient. I say "within reason" because there is no absolute protection against fraud. Transgressions may continue to occur, though probably with no greater frequency than now, but privacy will be protected.

There is no a priori reason for charges to be linked to clinical information once the charges leave the clinical facility. Charges can be separated from clinical content within the walls of hospitals, clinics, and offices. I am suggesting a standardized stratification system that would group charges by a new coding scheme, on the basis of mutually agreed-upon costs for preventive, diagnostic, and therapeutic measures. These charge codes, separated from their clinical antecedents, would then be sent on to the third-party payer.

With my plan, provisions would be established for internal review by staff members of the clinical facility to ensure the accuracy of the linkage between charge and procedure. And equally important, provisions would be established for external review by independent auditors. These could be chosen from respected members of the medical and business communities, who would visit the clinical facility to ensure the legitimacy of the charges, with scrutiny for accuracy, fairness, and honesty. Or, as Virgil Slee has suggested, financial auditing could be done by a certified public accounting firm, much the way a corporation is audited for its financial affairs. (Accounting firms would be liable for prosecution if they were to divulge confidential corporate information.) If the auditors certify that the clinic's records tell the truth, this would be accepted. If not, the charges would be adjusted within the clinical facility. But no confidential information would leave the facility unless under the direction of the patient or an authorized surrogate.

In managed care plans based on capitation, meaning that the insurer pays a fixed amount regardless of the care given individual patients, there is even less reason for the payer to have access to confidential medical information. If the costs to the clinic are higher than the allocated amount, the managed care company will *not* make up the difference. Yet currently, the companies insist on obtaining clinical information, the ICD-9 diagnostic codes at a minimum, for each patient in their plan.

Furthermore, there is potential risk to the patient with reimbursement based on capitation. When budgets are thus restricted, the financial incentive is to have more patients but do less for each patient seen. The clinician is under pressure to cut corners; efficiency sometimes takes precedence over quality. When capitation is implemented, therefore, there should be provision for peer review and audit to ensure that there are sufficient funds to cover reasonable medical costs for good medical care (with sufficient funds held in reserve in the event of emergencies), as well as to verify the accuracy, fairness, and honesty of the accounting. With my plan, information about the facility's medical finances would be readily available to the paying company for its use in negotiating subsequent contractual arrangements for payment, but no medical information would leave the hospital or clinic without the consent of the patient or the patient's representative.

The Naysayers

The third-party payers will ask, and already have, how they can trust hospitals, clinics, and clinicians to give accurate and honest accounting. They will argue that they are paying the bills and have a right to know what they are paying for. But we can remind them that they are using *our* money to pay the bills, and they are making a profit. Let us remember that until now, the trust has gone in one direction, toward the third-party payer. It is time for them to give their trust in return.

The third-party payers might ask, and already have, who will authorize the use of services; who will approve the plan for patient care. My answer is straightforward. When it comes to the payer practicing medicine, my prescription is to disallow it. The payers do not need to know the clinical information associated with charges for an individual patient. As things stand now, the financial conflict of interest and the trust that goes with it are heavily weighted in favor of the third-party payer. Let us reverse the process. Let us return the trust to the patient and clinician. Let auditing be done by a small group of disinterested peers, who would serve with the consent of all parties involved.

Third-party payers might argue, and already have, that I am indulging in what some have called the leisure of the theory class. Clearly, there will be hurdles along the way, and there are details of my plan to be worked out. But think of the advantages. Privacy would be protected. No legislation would be needed. There would be fewer data to process, and money would be saved—by the clinics and taxpayers, if not the third-party payers. And we would not have to investigate the Medical Insurance Bureau. It would disappear on its own, with disuse atrophy.

PART THREE

Modern Times

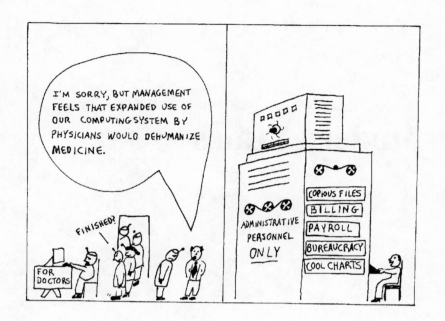

CHAPTER ELEVEN

Barriers to Cybermedicine

I f the computer is to become more widely available and useful as a patient's assistant—helping patients and their families maintain better health, manage medical problems when they occur, seek and use health care facilities in an enlightened manner, and participate as partners with clinicians in medical decisions—good materials must be written and tested. And progress is being made. Already there are good programs on PCs, such as those developed by David Gustafson, Patricia Brennan, and their coworkers to help patients with problems such as breast cancer and AIDS and by Lawrence Van Cura to help people assess various risks to their health. I hope the emphasis in the future will be on truly interactive health-related programs that capitalize on the power of the Internet and are available to all who have the capacity to go on-line—programs that are kept current and address the individual needs of the people who use them, with pictures and sound as well as text. The rate-limiting enzyme in the development of these programs, to use a biological metaphor, is one of resources. Well-written, informative, interactive medical materials are difficult and expensive to prepare, and the question is how best to support their development. Fortunately, however, few administrative barriers block the way of progress. The barriers are primarily financial, and these can be overcome with pressure from the patient in the role of consumer.

Good computing for the clinician in the hospital is another matter. As I have pointed out, there is often more useful computing for the doctor outside the hospital, on the Internet. Why? Why do so many American hospitals, clinics, and private offices have little or no computing that helps the doctor care for patients? The reasons are both real and imaginary. Let us consider the imaginary reasons first.

IMAGINARY BARRIERS TO CYBERMEDICINE

There is a tendency to assume that to introduce a computer to medicine is to introduce new, important clinical information that clinicians *should* acquire, and to assume that whether clinicians use the computer is a measure of their willingness and ability to master new technology. When terminals go unused, the explanation is sought in characteristics of the user, such as age, computer phobia, and lack of computer literacy, rather than characteristics of the computer programs, such as how well they work to help the clinician or patient.

Age and Computer Phobia

Blaming the already beleaguered clinician for being too old or computer phobic is a handy approach for computer manufacturers, systems analysts, and program developers whose programs are disliked and little used. This argument is reminiscent of the way automobile manufacturers used to blame drivers rather than defects in their cars until Ralph Nader set the record straight with *Unsafe at Any Speed*. When computer manufacturers ask, "How can we get physicians to use computers?" they are more likely to mean, "How can we get physicians to buy computers?" A better question would be, "How can we make our computers helpful?" Howard Bleich and I have a theorem that the quality of any computer program is *inversely* proportionate to the size of the manual sitting next to the terminal.

In our experience, age and computer phobia are unimportant as deterrents to the use of cybermedicine. In an informal study at Beth Israel Hospital in 1982, well before the widespread proliferation of personal computers, we found that staff physicians—who were older and presumably more prone to computer phobia than the medical students and house officers—were nevertheless equally well disposed toward the cybermedicine system and its helpfulness in patient care.

The same can be said for the population in general. With the advent of the Internet, millions of people are going on-line, undeterred by age or computer phobia. Computer phobia disappears rapidly when the machine is easy to use and helpful; and it has been amply demonstrated that people from three to ninety-three can use computers to their advantage.

Computer Literacy

Nor is lack of computer literacy an important barrier. People catch on quickly once they are able to try their hand. They don't need to know the inner workings of a machine to use it with good purpose. The belief that they do is an all-too-common misconception.

For the most part it is true that the person who invents a machine and understands its inner workings is also its first user. The early automobiles—Nicholas Joseph Cugnot's steam vehicle of the 1760s and Karl Benz's gasoline-powered carriage of the 1880s—were first operated by those who designed and built them. Almost certainly, Blaise Pascal was the first to use his mechanical adding machine (in the 1640s), Gottfried Leibniz the first to use his four-function mechanical calculator (in the 1670s), and William Burroughs the first to use his business machine (in the 1890s). Had Charles Babbage ever actually built his digital computer (in the 1820s), he would for sure have been the only person who knew how to use it. And so it has been with the more modern vacuum-tube and solid-state machines, with programming languages, and with the programs themselves.

Once a machine is in general use, however, it is no longer necessary for the user to understand its inner workings. Most of us drive our automobiles without knowing the theoretical foundations of the internal combustion engine; most of us use our telephones without understanding information theory, and turn on our electric lights without Ohm's law in mind.

So it has been with cybermedicine. During the first two decades of the use of computers in medicine (the 1950s and 1960s), those of us who wanted to use a computer typically had to program it ourselves, often in machine language. Programming in machine language (with instructions that are executed directly by the computer, one by one, without first being interpreted or compiled into simpler units) entails some understanding of the machine's inner workings. (Our programs with the LINC were written in machine language.) In the 1970s, most of us who used computers were still doing our own programming. We had higher-level languages (compilers and interpreters) and programming was easier for us, but we were still in close touch with the machine.

Now, of course, things have changed. Clinicians who know nothing about the inner workings of their computers can, to good advantage, use programs written by others. With a few simple keystrokes (though as yet in relatively few institutions, unfortunately), they can look up the results of diagnostic studies, get advice on patient care, search the medical literature, and communicate with each other by e-mail. Personal computers provide word processing and spreadsheet accounting programs that require little more understanding of the machine than how to turn it on. And of course, doctors and patients are using the Internet with increasing regularity.

Still, the idea that the doctor (or anyone else) must know the theoretical underpinnings of the computer—must be "computer literate"—to use the machine lingers on. This notion is kept alive in part by well-meaning, influential medical school academics, typically nonusers themselves, who are unnecessarily embarrassed by their own inexperience with computers and who believe, misguidedly, that an in-depth knowledge of computational theory is a prerequisite for productive use.

Then there are those persistent professors, often erstwhile programmers themselves, who want a computer course (required) to be part of the medical school curriculum. They want their students to be computer literate. They forget that most undergraduates are heavy users of the Internet and word processing (if not on their own machines, on machines provided by their colleges or universities), before they ever get to medical school, and that many doctors (particularly nonacademics) who have never taken a course in computing already use personal computers to good advantage without worrying about computer literacy.

If a medical student *wants* to know the theory behind a machine (be it a computer or an autoanalyzer), there should be facilities within the school to encourage this. But when curricula are already full, when even clinical courses such as pediatrics and obstetrics are themselves sometimes electives, the argument for a required course in computing is unconvincing. Neither clinicians nor patients need be computer literate, in the sense of understanding the inner workings of the machine, to use the computer in the practice of medicine.

Turn with me then, if you will, to some of the real obstacles that keep computers from serving the medical community effectively.

REAL BARRIERS TO CYBERMEDICINE

With cybermedicine for the clinician, the forces of bureaucracy play a prominent role. The impediment to good computing is more managerial, administrative, political, and territorial than technical or medical. And doctors are partly responsible. In the early days of the computer, they suspected that the machines would encroach on the practice of medicine rather than enhance it. By the time they understood that computers would not destroy the art of medicine, the opportunity to influence the computing in their hospitals and clinics was largely out of their hands.

The Administrator

There are two types of librarian in my experience: the one who wants you to take out the book and the one who doesn't. The former welcomes signs of use, signs that you have read and enjoyed the book. The latter worries that you might tear the pages, get food on the cover, or break the binding. The administrative goals of the institution determine which librarian will prevail. If the primary goal is to promote usage, it will be the former. If the primary goal is to protect inventory, it will be the latter.

In a like manner, there are two types of hospital administrator: the one who is both willing and able to help the clinician care for the patient and the one who isn't. The former wants to make it as easy as possible for the clinician to practice good medicine, wants to say yes to requests for help, even when this entails flexibility, ingenuity, and conscience. The latter is much more comfortable saying no. (Flexibility, ingenuity, and conscience are administratively risky.) Which administrator will prevail is again determined by goals. If the primary goal is to promote patient care, it will be Type 1; if the primary goal is to protect administrative order, it will be Type 2.

My first real-time experience with hospital bureaucracy was back in 1962 at Clark Air Force Base in the Philippines, where I served as a neurologist for two years. During medical school, internship, and residency, I had been isolated from hospital administrators, who were few in number in those days (typically *one* vice president per teaching hospital, if you can believe it). But at Clark Hospital—a group of M*A*S*H-like Quonset huts—it was different. Medical Service Corps officers—the forerunners of the vice-presidential administrators and middle managers that now pervade American hospitals—were all about us. And for the most part they were Type 2 administrators—en route to becoming functionaries with neither imagination nor conscience (as Abba Eban once described the tax collectors of Mesopotamia). They would get to the hospital at nine in the morning, leave promptly at five, and dress in proper uniform, but whatever role they played in patient care served for the most part to *impede* the process.

An Administrative Formula

Not all administrators at Clark were Type 2, mind you. There were some Type 1s who really wanted to help, but they were in the minority. Also, they were mostly of lower rank—typically lieutenants or sergeants. For example, my staff sergeant—Sgt. Rulebender—could really get things done. In fact, the doctors there, who were very busy (the Vietnam War was escalating) and doing their best to practice good medicine, noticed an interesting phenomenon among the administrators: the higher their rank, the lower their competence (that is, their ability and willingness to help). With homage to C. Northcote Parkinson, I formalized this as an inverse proportion:

$$C \text{ (COMPETENCE)} = 1/R \text{ (RANK)}$$

This is not to be confused with the "Peter principle," which pertains to people who continue to be promoted because they *are* competent until they reach a position in which they are incompetent, where they then remain. The dynamics of $C = 1/R$ were to become increasingly clear to me as I learned about the process of military promotion.

At the end of each two-year period, the Medical Service Corps officer would receive what was called an "efficiency rating"—on a scale of "poor" to "outstanding"—from his (they were all men) superior officer, who was another administrator. Accordingly, the administrator's allegiance belonged to the administrator who would rate him, not to the doctors, whom he could displease without risk. Because it is virtually impossible to make a good suggestion without implying a criticism—why didn't the superior officer think of it himself?—suggestions were not well received. Hence, the fewer the suggestions about how to help the doctors and their patients, the higher the efficiency rating. And promotion depended on a rating of "outstanding." Accordingly, as the administrator rose in rank he became decreasingly willing and able himself and increasingly threatened by suggestions from subordinates (which in turn dampened their enthusiasm for making any). By the time the administrator made bird colonel, the process was complete: He was now a functionary with neither imagination nor conscience.

C = 1/R in Civilian Life

My career in the military ended after the usual two-year stint, but I have no reason to believe that $C = 1/R$ is less apt today than it was in the 1960s. And I know for sure that it applies increasingly well to civilian hospitals—with their corporate ranking systems, such as manager, director, assistant vice president, vice president, chief financial officer (CFO), together with the chief information officer (CIO), chief operating officer (COO), and chief executive officer (CEO)—where Type 2 administrators are proliferating. They are hired, promoted, and fired by other administrators, to whom they give their allegiance. Hence there is little administrative incentive for them to help the doctors. Type 2s are assisted in their pursuit of administrative orderliness by the currently popular view (promulgated by a surprising number of business schools) that the less the administrator knows about the specific business, the better will be the management. (Imagine a Type 2 administrator in the role of "vice president for *clinical services*"! Next hospital, please.)

The Type 2 gives much more importance, much more status to managerial position than to technical competence. Competence is high-risk for the Type 2, something to be kept in check—"No creative people in the inner office, thank you." The Type 2 is uncomfortable in the presence of people with tangible skills, such as the computer programmer, the engineer, the scientist, and the clinician (clinicians are a necessary evil at best in the Type 2 mind-set—"if only they could be done away with, but then . . . "). Only managers are welcome in Type 2 meetings. Albert Einstein would never get promoted in the Type 2 environment.

There are still some exceptional hospitals in the United States where Type 1 administrators predominate, and I have been fortunate to work in them and with the Type 1 administrators in the CCC. But I am afraid I must say their numbers are on the wane. The current trend toward the corporatizing of the American hospital can only accentuate the process.

It should be pointed out that competence in my equation is defined from the perspective of the clinician, not the administrator; surely, there are Type 2 administrators who believe that their process of promotion is based on merit. The promotion of the Type 2 administrator, therefore, should not be confused with the well-known situation—the reverse of the Peter principle if you will—in which an incompetent civil servant who cannot be fired is promoted as a means of good riddance. Nor should it be confused with the "Dilbert principle," whereby the administrator is promoted to a position of harmlessness. The Type 2 administrator is *not* harmless.

Cybermedicine is still not high among the priorities of the Type 2 CFOs and CIOs who control the computer rooms in so many of our hospitals and clinics. If the financial computing systems get the bills out more or less on time, their jobs are secure, and the board of directors is pleased.

The Committee

As it is with the administrator, so it is with the committee. There is the Type 1, with a well-defined goal, a few members, and a short life span—a committee whose work is judged by outcome. And there is the Type 2, with an ill-defined goal, a lot of members, and an infinite life span, whose work is judged by form and process.

Committees are at the foundation of most institutions, whether they are academic, medical, industrial, or governmental. All colleges and universities, for example, must have at least two of them: the admissions committee for students and the promotions committee for faculty. But I doubt that there has ever been an institution of any size with only two committees on its premises. The reason is that the committee is self-propagating; like Parkinson's "officials" or Type 2 administrators—who proliferate exponentially, regardless of the job to be done—the committee assumes a reproductive life of its own.

The explanation for this phenomenon, though perhaps not immediately apparent, is straightforward: it is more prestigious to *form* a committee than to serve on one. The most prestigious committee-related behavior, typically reserved for the president, governor, chancellor, or CEO, is to form a committee but attend no meetings—"the CEO's Sitting Committee on Management Information Systems," for example, reminiscent of Her Majesty's Ship, which she never boards.

A somewhat less prestigious committee-related move, typically reserved for the COO, CFO, or an administrator of equivalent rank, is to form a committee—"standing" as it is sometimes referred to—put in a perfunctory appearance, tell the members about the momentous nature of their mission, and then disappear to be seen no more. But what about those who must actually serve on a committee and attend its meetings?

For those who must serve, the best role by far is that of chair, one of whom was the now-forgotten genius who, in the primordial era of institutions, conceived of a way to keep his personal committee meetings to a minimum and at the same time enhance his prestige: he invented the subcommittee—and formed two of them. He knew that there must be at least two subcommittees. A single subcommittee might resemble the standing committee and be confused with it, undermining the committee chair's prestige rather than enhancing it. The newly appointed chairs of the two subcommittees—those who understand the process, that is—each move quickly to form two of their own—sub-subcommittees. And so it goes, with sub-sub-sub-committees giving birth to sub-sub-sub-subcommittees, and on and on. Imagine a rising pyramid of committees, proliferating in a manner independent of whatever ostensible purpose the standing committee was supposed to serve.

It should be mentioned here that I know people in a number of institutions (and it is likely that you do as well) who actually *like* to go to meetings, who welcome the opportunity to serve on committees or subcommittees at any level, and who always respond to the chair's closing question—"Is there any other issue to discuss?"—with another issue. These people, of course, augment the proliferation of committees and their progeny. But for those of you who don't like committees yet must serve on them (your job may depend on it), here are a few tips that may prove useful: (1) Avoid subcommittees at all costs. (2) Never accept a writing assignment. More than likely, the assignment is a gambit to transfer responsibility (read "onus") to your shoulders. Now the chair will be waiting for you; *you* will be the one who is slowing things down. If you pass the chair in the hall, you will feel guilty; if things go wrong, it will be your fault. And whatever you finally do write will go unread, laid to rest in the filing cabinet of the person who formed the committee. (If it is bulk that is needed, offer to clear your desk.) (3) Fortify yourself with a self-beeper for use when there is no hope of an early closure. And (4) skip one meeting. If there are no repercussions, try a sliding-scale approach; first (at random) skip a meeting a month, next (judiciously) skip two meetings a month, then (with caution) three, and finally (de facto) resign. You may never be missed. Now maybe you can get some work done.

Type 2 committees and their subcommittee offspring are pervading hospitals and clinics at an alarming rate. With the Type 2 CFO or CIO in charge, the committee is yet another formidable barrier to good cybermedicine. The more committees there are, the more meetings to attend. When you are always in a meeting, it's hard to find time to do much computing.

The Company

Vendors of hospital computing systems usually try to sell their products to the CEO, COO, CFO, or CIO, to one of the hospital's growing cadre of executive, senior, associate, or assistant vice presidents, or to one of the rapidly proliferating senior, middle, or assistant departmental managers—*not* to a clinician. Accordingly, the programs sold and delivered are financial, managerial, or stand-alone departmental. They may come with the promise of cybermedicine, but they do not deliver. They may serve the needs of the buyer or department but for the most part are of little use to the clinician in the care of the patient.

If a company promises cybermedicine, it is important for the potential buyer to know whether the system is up and running somewhere, *anywhere,* and whether clinicians are using it. Yet information about usage is hard to come by. Data from companies that market computing systems are often unavailable or unreliable; it is difficult if not impossible to glean from these companies the extent to which someone, *anyone,* actually uses their systems. And of course keeping track of use is something that a computer can be readily programmed to do. Is there something these companies have to hide? Do their accomplishments not live up to their promises? Some time ago I saw a press release claiming that one hospital was using a commercial system with "more than 250 working stations . . . making it one of the world's largest patient data management systems." A telephone call to the hospital revealed that there had indeed been a purchase, but that most of the workstations had yet to be installed, and not one was in use.

The Cost

In the early days, capital investment in hardware was a major consideration in any decision about the type of computing a hospital or clinic would have. If the hospital had already purchased a large, expensive mainframe computer for fiscal purposes, then clinical programs, if they were to be implemented, were expected to run on the same machine, even though it was not well suited to these programs. This is no longer the case. Many hospitals and clinics can now afford to replace their overpriced, cumbersome mainframes with networks of inexpensive and flexible minicomputers. They can, that is, if the forces of bureaucracy can be overcome. The cost of cybermedicine software will still be formidable but should be well within the range of what most hospitals now pay for their managerial and financial computing systems.

The Consultant

And then there is the consultant. But this should have its own chapter.

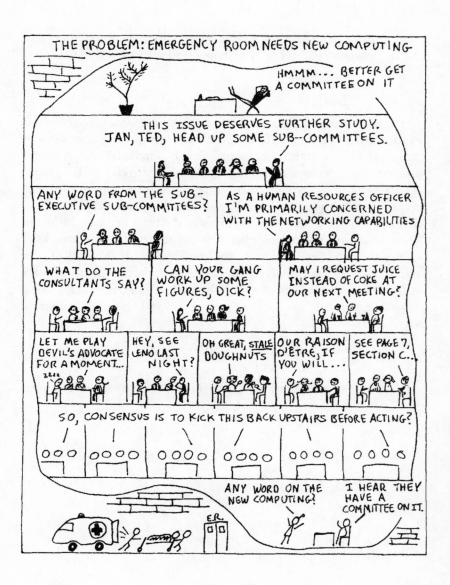

CHAPTER TWELVE

The Importance of
Being Ernst

T hese are good times for consultants. Long-established companies are merging and branching out. Firms such as Price-waterhouseCoopers, Deloitte & Touche, Peat Marwick, Accenture (formerly Arthur Andersen), and Ernst & Young, whose services were once limited to accounting and auditing, are now in the business of selling advice, even to hospitals and clinics. Hospitals and clinics are especially good business. Their CEOs, CFOs, COOs, and CIOs are popular targets. Just as Dylan Thomas's uncles were always there at Christmas in Wales, consultants are always there at conferences on medical computing, replete with booths. And now, in a remarkable process of metastatic proliferation, consultants permeate hospitals and their computing centers.

Not all hospital consultants are bad, of course. There are two types, just as there are two types of administrator. Type 1 is experienced, knowledgeable, and forthright, offering constructive criticism and recommendations even if the advice is unwelcome. Type 1 wants to get the job done and move on to new challenges. Type 2, on the other hand, prefers to charge by the day, and does *not* want to move on. A principal strategy of the Type 2 consultant is to figure out what the paying client wants to hear, and then take as long as possible to say it. A principal function of the Type 2 is to bolster the client's ego and off-load responsibility for risky decisions.

Type 2 consulting companies are staffed by what consultologists call *finders, minders,* and *grinders.* Finders are senior vice presidents whose job is to reel in the clients. Minders are middle managers who aspire to be finders, and whose job is to mind the grinders. And grinders are freshly graduated MBAs without previous experience, whose job is to do the consulting.

With as much delay as possible, a minder, who has had little experience with cybermedicine (and, of course, has not read *Cybermedicine*), identifies the *real* experts in the client's institution, who could themselves become good, Type 1 consultants and charge for their expertise, but are obligated by managerial decree—their jobs might depend on it—to share their experience with the consultant. It is the grinder's job then to interview these people. Thus, while the company is being lucratively remunerated, the grinder, on the road to promotion, can soak up a little of the experts' knowledge and pass this on to the minder and finder for use in landing future clients—learning on the job at the client's expense. A good deal, if you can get away with it.

Dickens once observed that the one great principle of the law is to make business for itself. In this regard, I see a parallel between the Type 2 lawyer (the subject of another book) and the Type 2 consultant. By way of illustration, let me turn to a short parable. You may think you recognize some of the characters, but of course any resemblance to actual persons, living or dead, is purely coincidental.

REINVENTING REORGANIZATION (A PARABLE FOR MODERN TIMES)

I was to learn that [managers] tend to meet any new situation by reorganizing, and the wonderful method it can be for creating the illusion of progress while producing confusion, inefficiency, and demoralization.

—Attributed to Petronius Arbiter, 66 A.D.

In the beginning, physicians were wary of computers. They were more than willing to leave the big machines alone, out of sight in the fiscal department, safely removed from the practice of medicine. By the time physicians realized that computers might actually help with patient care, territorial imperatives had been firmly established: the CFO and the CIO had control of the computer—and the large budget needed to support it—and were not about to give these up. Like space and parking, the computer had become an important source of managerial control. And to this day, in most American hospitals and clinics, the CFO and CIO control the computer room—and clinical programs are not high on their list of priorities.

In one hospital, however, things are different. Suburban Hospital, a West Coast teaching hospital, has a cybermedicine system, developed by a talented group of computer programmers, physicians, and engineers, together with a Type 1 administrator, Mr. Rulebender (now out of the Air Force), who has no title; there are no manuals. The system is self-instructional and easy to use. It transmits test results on request from authorized users, offers consultation on diagnosis and treatment, provides access to the MEDLINE database, has a heavily used e-mail system, does the financials, and supports the lean Type 1 administrative staff. It is regarded as a model and is heavily used by physicians, nurses, medical students, and other clinicians throughout the hospital, who send love letters to the computer by e-mail. The financial programs run as a by-product of the clinical systems, and the hospital's receivables are in excellent shape.

But now there is a change in management. Suburban Hospital merges with Paragon Healthcare, Inc. to form SubPar Health, a 501(c)(3) not-for-profit HMO and a wholly owned subsidiary of Mega Health, Inc., a for-profit conglomerate. The Type 2 administrators at SubPar are now in charge, and the days of cybermedicine are numbered.

In accordance with Parkinson's law ("An official wants to multiply subordinates, not rivals"), the new CEO, Chauncey Nurdstock, moves quickly to hire a raft of subordinates—ten senior vice presidents, each of whom appoints two vice presidents, each of whom hires two assistant vice presidents, and a new CFO, Mr. Martinet, recruited from Mega Health. Rulebender now reports to Martinet. (There is as yet no CIO.) Martinet doesn't like Rulebender—he is not a company man; he doesn't believe in organizational charts; he allocates too much of the hospital's computing to the doctors (Martinet doesn't like doctors, either); he doesn't understand that computing should be governed by financial needs, not patient care; he doesn't show the proper respect; and his irreverent attitude is hardly amusing. Martinet can't say these things out loud, of course. "Rulebender can't manage," is the best he can do.

Martinet, on the advice of Nurdstock (who doesn't like Rulebender, either), determines to recruit a CIO. He turns to a headhunter (who also consults) out of Denver who recruits our old friend Mr. Binary from Midwest University Hospital. Binary's application has been held in strictest confidence at his request, in case he should decide to stay put at Midwest Hospital. His track record at Midwest is not discussed; it is understood that Martinet will make discrete inquiries.

A Type 1 administrator at Midwest, who has been looking for a way to get rid of Binary, takes Martinet's telephone call with barely suppressed joy. At Midwest there is chaos in the computing center, serious financial problems, and no computing for doctors despite millions spent. Yet Midwestman's candor prevails, and he gives Binary a less-than-glowing recommendation. To Martinet, however, this news is not unwelcome. He likes to surround himself with people less competent than he, in keeping with another of Parkinson's tenets. They don't threaten him; they put him in a good light. Martinet interviews Binary and takes to him right off. "Just the man I've been looking for," he is heard to say.

Once on site, Binary is eager to rid himself of the cybermedicine computing system and install one with his own stamp on it. On the recommendation of Nurdstock, who occupies the oak-paneled executive suite down the hall next to Martinet's (cherry paneled), Binary approaches S&S (Skimpole & Skimpole), an accounting firm in Boston that has branched out to medical consulting, whose knowledge of the consulting game is exceeded only by its ignorance of computers in medicine.

Two senior finders at S&S smell blood. They fly into town for the first meeting, held in the boardroom of their regional office. (Finders always fly *into* town for the first meeting, even if they have to fly *out* of town in order to fly back.) Nurdstock, Martinet, and Binary are impressed. The hook is set. In the oak-paneled boardroom, over juice, coffee, and Danish, the sales pitch begins. There are introductory comments from the finders, followed by a well-worn stock spiel from three minders—an hour-long series of flow charts, flip charts, and screen shots replete with bullets and arrowheads. Nurdstock, Martinet, and Binary can't follow the presentation (which, in fact, is unencumbered by meaning); they just sit there and nod knowingly, hoping to think of a question or two to ask that might impress the finders, who are about to rush back to the airport.

The fish is landed before the hour is up. A seven-figure contract is signed. But for S&S this is a loss leader; the *real* money will come later.

Phase I

SubPar hosts a wine-and-cheese party to introduce its staff to S&S (a finder flies in to offer a few words of congratulation). A minder and five grinders arrive on site, and Phase I is launched. The first item on the agenda is to form a task force. More grinders arrive with their minders, in a ratio of 5:1. Gestational proliferation is under way. The task force spawns a sitting committee, which in turn spawns two standing committees, which in turn spawn four subcommittees, which in turn spawn eight sub-subcommittees, some chaired by Binary, some by S&S minders, and some by their grinders. Sixteen workshops are scheduled during the first month. The minders and their grinders, some of whom are now full-time at SubPar (S&S is downsizing but will hire them back if necessary), go from one meeting to the next. Cybermedicine staff are required to attend all meetings; computer maintenance grinds to a halt.

Phase II

S&S issues its standard interim report, glossy and laced with consultantspeak: "data warehouse," "closed systems," "open systems," "connectivity," "interface engine," and "leverage." In the tradition of S&S's in-house corporate parsimony, the report is prepared in boilerplate, designed for use in virtually any client hospital; only the names need be changed. The prose, designed to appeal to Nurdstock, Martinet, and Binary, contains no surprises (*the good parasite does not destroy the host*). In summary, the report recommends "reengineering" and "facilitation," with emphasis on "leveraging" and "prioritizing." Give the financials the highest priority (the clinicals can wait); develop an organizational chart; institute a formidable number of regulations (for example, "Physicians Are Not Allowed in the Computing Room"). And as soon as Binary and his committees complete the organizational chart, they should plan on downsizing (from among the technically competent, it is implied, particularly those who also speak their minds;

S&S will help), and upsizing (there is always a need for more Type 2s). Focus groups for the remaining staff will be in order.

The report continues. Binary should replace the "legacy" cyber-medicine system with a "best-of-breed" "data repository," purchased from a large, well-known company whose product is mostly fiscal in function. The computing will be expensive to buy, hard to install, and cumbersome if not impossible to operate. (This ensures the need for continuous consultation, with S&S on retainer, which is part of the recommendation.) Bison Computing, Inc., meets all the requirements and is the vendor of choice.

Mr. Rulebender, now relegated to co-chair of a sub-sub-sub committee, sees the handwriting on the wall and leaves. The computing deteriorates noticeably, and there is discontent among the clinicians. But Nurdstock, Martinet, and Binary promise new and better things in the future. "Rulebender couldn't manage and was out of touch with new technology," they advise the clinicians.

Phase III

SubPar signs long-term contracts with S&S and Bison Computing, which has agreed to "transition" some of its own consultants to help those from S&S. (There is a rumor of a financial arrangement between Bison and S&S.) "Risks and benefits will be shared," Binary proclaims. (A careful look at the contract would reveal that SubPar will be taking the risks, and Bison and S&S will share the benefits. But Binary doesn't look; he is busy reorganizing his organizational chart.)

With a grinder by his side, Binary prepares memos for distribution, "dictated but not signed." He hires ten directors, each of whom hires two assistant directors, each of whom hires two managers. Now seventy of the rectangular boxes on Binary's organizational chart, replete with interconnecting lines, have names in them (eighty to go, once all the assistant managers are hired). New minders and grinders arrive. "It takes a lot of managers to downsize," Binary is heard to say.

Phase IV

What downsizing occurs is from the ranks of those who do the computing. As the management staff grows, there are fewer and fewer programmers and engineers to be managed. Reluctant to take orders from grinders, doers follow Rulebender out the door to organizations where competence is still rewarded. "Have you seen *The Titanic?*" one programmer asks another on their way out the door. "At least they had music going down," comes the reply.

In the meantime, Bison Computing has yet to get its machines up and running, and the doctors at SubPar are worried. They can't find the results of their lab tests, and nothing happens when they turn on their high-resolution, multifaceted graphics terminals. (One bemused clinician calls the newly formed "help desk" and is told, "Sorry, I can't help you.") They try to e-mail Binary, but the new e-mail system is inoperative. They march to Binary's office to badger him for help.

This puts Binary in a bit of a bind. For one thing, he is not well versed in the subject of cybermedicine. For another, it is becoming clear, even to him, that the Bison computers will have limited function, *if* they are ever turned on—something called matrix accounting, at best. Even Nurdstock and Martinet are getting antsy. *Something must be done.*

A minder, by way of a grinder, gives Binary his next move: another committee, standing, anointed by Nurdstock, announced by Martinet, and co-chaired by Binary and the grinder, with a middle manager from Bison (now on SubPar's payroll) as member, ex officio. They should also appoint a token doctor and a token nurse to the committee (the first medical input since the arrival of S&S).

At the first meeting, Grinder, whose sole clinical experience was a tonsillectomy at age five, reminds those in attendance, including the doctor and nurse (with forty years of clinical experience between *them*), that the patient comes first. Grinder and Binary then hand out reorganizational charts—ten pages of rectangular boxes with interconnecting lines—and announce with pride that they have gotten rid of the last of the legacy programs and have signed a contract for more computers from Bison. Mr. Bison, speaking for the first time and with the help of overheads, announces how pleased he is that his company, with its new line of Super Megasaurs, is now in a position to put SubPar in the forefront of hospital computing. Then Grinder speaks for thirty-five minutes about the conversion of the hospital's financial programs to the new matrix billing system, replete with packages, client servers, open architecture, and connectivity—"In other words," he declares with pride, "We will have a best-of-breed data warehouse." The token doctor and token nurse don't know what this means, but they don't ask. They don't want to prolong the meeting. "Content-free," mumbles the nurse to the doctor on her way out.

At the next meeting, Grinder transfers the onus for cybermedicine to the doctor and nurse with a writing assignment: "Document your needs in a memo," and asks each of them to serve as members on one of two newly formed subcommittees, "Director in Charge of Clinical Services," Grinder's new title, chair. Grinder follows up the meeting with a memo of his own, "dictated but not signed," stressing the importance of detailed documentation prepared in advance. In the meantime, the few remaining Type 1s disappear from the financial office and computing center, the computing continues to deteriorate, and the financial situation goes from bad to worse.

Clinical Refugees

The token doctor is increasingly concerned, as is the token nurse, the token pharmacist, and the token technologist. They have documented and redocumented their requests, but still they have no computing. They threaten to resign from the standing committee as well as the subcommittee. In response, Grinder and Binary convene another meeting. Bison is the featured speaker. He presents the plans for a new total hospital information system (HIS), Megasaur-based, together with a management information system (MIS), both integral components of best-of-breed information technology (IT) and in the forefront of information systems (IS). What he means, of course, is yet more hardware, a bigger budget, another cumbersome, partially working, multi-matrixed billing system, and an expansion of the contract with S&S. The doctor and nurse are not reassured.

But no matter, Binary and Martinet are pleased, as is Nurdstock, when informed by memo, "dictated *and* signed"; they have something to announce. They schedule a wine-and-cheese reception to honor HIS and MIS; they invite all the administrators (exclusively Type 2, by now), all the people from S&S and Bison (including the regional vice president for sales at Bison), and as an afterthought, the token doctor and token nurse. Later, to save money, Nurdstock and Martinet do some more downsizing, cutting back on nurses, pharmacists, laboratory technologists, and phlebotomists, and transfer their responsibilities to the remaining nurses and house officers, who are too tired to protest.

At the suggestion of Minder, delivered by Grinder, Binary gets Bison's updated versions of HIS and MIS (HIS-U and MIS-U), hires ten more assistant managers, is promoted to senior vice president, and has his office refurbished in cherry wood. Martinet is promoted to COO and has his office oak paneled. Binary and Martinet are now above the fray, so to speak. A sign on Binary's desk reads, "The buck never *gets* here." (Grinder is appointed CIO, and Minder becomes CFO, acting. It's now *their* job to stay the critics.) Priorities are once again in administrative order.

But the doctors, nurses, and patients are *not* pleased. patient care is suffering.

Phase V

This is the S&S flak-catching phase. It is understood that Nurdstock, Martinet, and Binary will blame S&S for SubPar's situation, and they do. This protects management and has little effect on the consultants from S&S, who with the timing of good snake oil salesmen have already left town.

But SubPar's days are numbered. The doctors and nurses take their patients elsewhere. The financial outlook is bleak. No loans can be secured. No Type 1s are there to help. At the point of terminus, there is one patient, suspended in semianimated coma à la Robin Cook, surrounded by a thousand administrators. Shortly thereafter, SubPar closes its doors.

Nurdstock and Binary take senior positions with Bison Computing, and Martinet is now a finder with S&S, hooking new clients. Rulebender has formed his own company (very lean on administrators and administrative titles), and has installed good cybermedicine in several consultant-free hospitals.

—⁓—

What then does the future hold for us? Are we destined to follow Nurdstock, Martinet, Binary, Bison, Finder, Minder, and Grinder down the garden path? Or can we join forces with Rulebender?

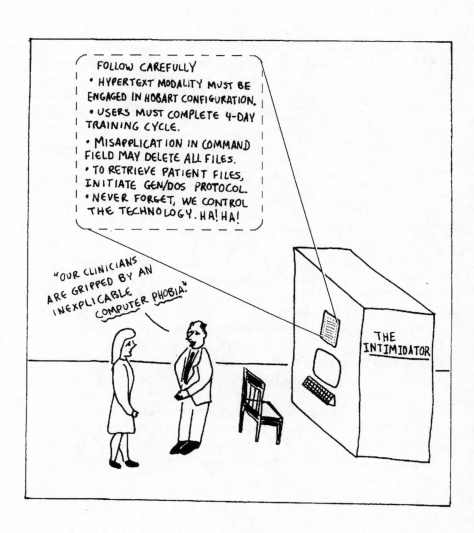

CHAPTER THIRTEEN

New Horizons

I t used to be that one of the rewards of being a doctor was being your own boss. Today, however, most doctors work for other people. As a political force within hospitals and clinics, doctors and other clinicians are poorly organized. The few who do demand good cybermedicine are likely to find themselves on a sub (or sub-sub) committee, token members dutifully accepting their writing assignments. "Write me a memo" is the administrative mechanism by which nothing gets done.

For their part, patients commonly believe that the computer is in fact being used to its full capacity in hospitals and clinics. This misconception is promulgated by those members of the computing industry who advertise total hospital and management information systems that are neither total nor clinically informative. It is also promulgated by Type 2 consultants, for whom prophecy is a substitute for accomplishment, and who will promise almost anything as long as a lucrative consulting contract is in the offing.

WHAT THE CLINICIAN CAN DO

Doctors and patients may fail to be assertive about cybermedicine, but they do not suffer from computer phobia, or computer illiteracy, nor are they too old to use modern technology. A computer program that clinicians or patients prefer not to use probably offers no advantage over traditional methods of processing and presenting information. Young or old, accustomed to the keyboard or not, clinicians (and patients) will turn readily to a computer that is helpful.

But we clinicians must be more assertive. We must seek out the Type 1 administrators at our hospitals and clinics and convince them that good cybermedicine is in their own best interest—that it will increase efficiency and save money as well as improving patient care.

Those of us who do research on computer applications in medicine have a special responsibility in this regard: to see that the benefits that are possible and those that have already been achieved are brought to the attention of clinicians and administrators alike. In hospitals where computers are used primarily for fiscal purposes, what computer to buy and what software to use are viewed as financial decisions. When a CFO or CIO—officials all-too-rarely familiar with the practice of medicine—selects the hospital's computing system, the needs of clinicians and patients are typically not considered in the decision. If good cybermedicine is to prevail, clinicians must insist on participating meaningfully in the process of selecting systems for their hospitals. One of my goals is to remove medical computing from its administrative and financial domain and make it a medical discipline, analogous to radiology and clinical pathology, in the pursuit of improving patient care.

Once the computing industry learns that hospitals will accept nothing but the best possible cybermedicine, programs that truly help in the practice of medicine will become available in the marketplace.

QUESTIONS TO ASK

When the decisions about computing are being shared, when clinicians and administrators are working together to buy a cybermedicine system, they should first interview representatives of the prospective company. They should do this themselves, avoiding consultants and their vested interests. As a team, they must be willing to assume responsibility for the outcome of their decision, good or bad, and not pass this on to each other, to their colleagues, or to a hired scapegoat.

One strategy is to ask the company representative where the system is working best. (I've noticed that the site that is pointed to tends to be geographically remote from the point at which the question is asked; if you are in southern Florida, don't be surprised if the site is north of British Columbia.) Then call the hospital or clinic to verify that the system is in place. Then, if you possibly can, visit the hospital (be prepared for a long journey) and interview the users whom the system is designed to serve. It is important to speak with a user rather than the person who made the decision to buy, who is probably not a user and may be more interested in defending the purchase than in assessing its quality.

The questions to ask are straightforward: What are the capabilities of the system? Does the system record usage, and if not, why not? How often is the computing being used, and by whom? How well is the computing liked? What are the true costs of the system? What is the effect of the computer on the hospital's finances? And of course most important, what is its effect on patient care? If responses engender optimism, I would proceed. If not, I would turn to another company.

WHAT THE PATIENT CAN DO

The patient as well as the doctor should bring pressure to bear on the powers that be. Does your doctor have ready access by computer to the results of diagnostic studies, to advice and consultation, and to the medical literature? Does the computer serve to protect your privacy? If not, why not? It is your right to have good computing in your hospital and clinic.

If the computer is to be more fully used as a patient's assistant, in the home and other places of convenience, substantial resources must be devoted to the effort. As I have noted, however, there will be fewer administrative barriers than in hospitals and clinics. If patients, as consumers, purchasers, taxpayers, and voters, demand good cybermedicine on-line, I am optimistic that it will be forthcoming.

CLOSING THE LOOP
BETWEEN CLINICIAN AND PATIENT

First used primarily for communication between clinician and clinician and between patient and patient, teleconverse is now used increasingly to enable and enhance communication between clinician and patient. This is one of the most promising applications of cybermedicine, with patient and doctor interacting as peers on behalf of better medicine. E-mail, of course, is the most prevalent form of teleconverse. With its unique powers of reliable, asynchronous communication, e-mail is beginning to rival the telephone as a means of electronic patient-clinician dialogue. As more and more attention is given both to the risks and benefits of e-mail in medicine, early concerns on the part of clinicians about the potential misuse and overuse of e-mail are giving way to a better understanding of the good use of this powerful means of communication. In this light, Barbara Kane and Daniel Sands have compiled and published helpful suggestions for the use of e-mail between patient and clinician—*Guidelines for the Use of Patient-Centered E-Mail*—with consideration of confidentiality, privacy, propriety, and the law, as well as of medically related issues.

Telemedicine

Telemedicine is the name used for remote medical consultation with the use of pictures. Telemedicine by means of two-way television has been used for over twenty years, primarily in radiology, whereby a remotely located clinician could obtain a radiologist's interpretation of an X-ray on the spot, in real time. The technology has been expensive, however, and its use in medicine has been limited, for the most part, to helping doctors and nurses care for patients in sparsely populated rural areas. On the other hand, the costs of long-distance visual communication can be expected to go down substantially with more and more use of the Internet and the rapidly evolving technology of wireless communication.

Baby CareLink

As with other forms of teleconverse in medicine, which were used initially for communication between clinicians and between patients, computer-based telemedicine is now in early use for communication between clinician and patient. Baby CareLink, developed by James Gray, Charles Safran, and their colleagues in the CCC and the Department of Neonatology at Beth Israel Deaconess Medical Center, is such a program. It was designed for use by the families of very-low-birth-weight babies, babies who need special pediatric care and must be confined in a neonatal intensive care unit during the early days of life. Baby CareLink uses the Internet, Web technology, e-mail, and two-way television to enhance communication between the baby's family, in their home, and the staff of the neonatal unit in the hospital. The program offers the parents medical information and emotional support through verbal communication and visual contact. The parents can see their baby, observe the neonatal care, and converse with the staff about their baby's progress and how best to care for their baby once he or she goes home. As with medically related chat groups, Baby CareLink also offers a communication link to enable families of very-low-birth-weight babies to interact with each other. Early results with the program demonstrate that Baby CareLink improves the satisfaction of parents with their baby's neonatal care. Furthermore, results suggest that the program facilitates earlier discharge of babies to their homes by supporting the educational and emotional needs of the families. (Baby CareLink is now marketed by Clinician Support Technology, Inc., and I must mention here that I am a member of the medical advisory board and a part owner of this new company.)

PatientSite

In the tradition of patient-computer dialogue and patient power, John Halamka, David Rind, Daniel Sands, and their colleagues at Beth Israel Deaconess Medical Center and the CCC have created PatientSite, a Web site that provides patients with a means to communicate with their clinicians and to gain access to information in their medical records. With PatientSite, patients who have access to the Internet can request appointments, view upcoming appointments, view the results of laboratory tests and X-ray interpretations, view their lists of medications, and ask questions and receive explanations about their medical care as well as the charges for their medical care.

PatientSite was implemented on a trial basis in April 2000. Thus far, fifty physicians and over two thousand patients have enrolled in the project, and the numbers are growing. A formal evaluation of

PatientSite is under way, and preliminary results indicate that the program is working well, to the satisfaction of both patient and physician.

A DREAM FOR THE FUTURE

I have a modest dream for the future, my own indulgence in wishing as a substitute for doing. This is how I'd like medical care to be practiced when I become a patient.

—⁓—

Gradually with time, all medical services will move out of the hospital to places of convenience for the patient. The hospital as we know it today—ever larger, more corporate, and more bureaucratic—will disappear. It will be unnecessary to concern ourselves with Messrs. Nurdstock, Martinet, Binary, Finder, Minder, Grinder, Bison, and their corporate and administrative hierarchy. The clinical haven of the future (I call it the *clinhaven*) will be a decentralized facility, small and conveniently located within or adjacent to a residential area—urban, suburban, or rural—within walking distance for many patients. Stays in the clinhaven will be appropriate for the illness, and complex diagnostic and therapeutic procedures will be possible on an ambulatory basis.

The clinhaven will be staffed by skilled, humanistic clinicians, who also run the facility, with patients and prospective patients on the board of directors. Medical students will train in the clinhaven. Doctors will make house calls. Clinicians and patients will know each others' names and will work together as colleagues. Administrators, few in number and all Type 1s, will be available as needed. The atmosphere will be convivial. Waiting time will be short. Parking will be plentiful. Vans will be available for transportation to and from.

The clinhaven will be equipped with the latest in medical technology, including good cybermedicine. In design it will be more like a small local hospital than a mega medical center, but it will have all the necessary resources to provide comprehensive medical care.

There will be local governance and prepaid financing for major expenses, with provisions for patients who cannot pay for routine care. The quality of care will determine the financing, not the reverse. Confidentiality will be protected; *no* clinical information will be released to third-party payers, *whoever* they may be, without the patient's consent.

Much of medical care will then move back to the home. With tele-converse readily available for patient, prospective patient, and clinician alike, patients themselves will manage common, important medical problems, in ready communication with their doctors and other clinicians. Even complex laboratory tests, once solely in the province of the large medical center or commercial laboratory, will be done by the patient, with easy-to-use equipment available to the home. Costs will go down, and time will be saved. But most important, the quality of medical care will be high.

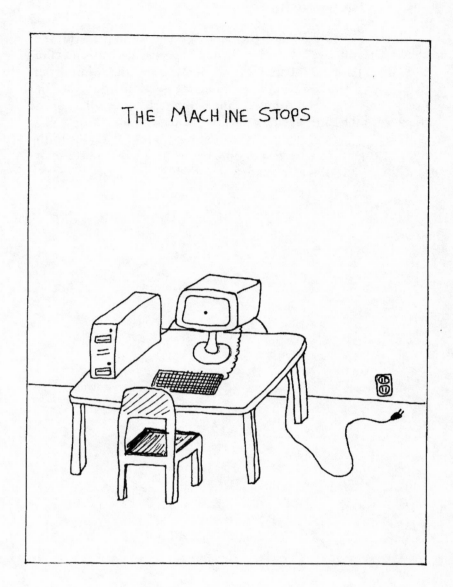

Epilogue

Alexis de Tocqueville once observed that Americans would do almost anything to avoid walking. On the way to town, for example, an American would wait an hour for a ride rather than walk the same distance in half the time. What the great French sociologist observed with bemusement in the nineteenth century would have boggled his mind in the twentieth. Automatic transportation is everywhere. Escalators, elevators, and moving walkways pervade our buildings, malls, and airports. In summertime, we can be seen shivering in place on our moving walkways in airtight enclosures, while fossil fuel is consumed to combat the energy of the sun. Outdoors, the sidewalk is absent from modern urban planning.

Those who visited the World's Fair in 1939 may recall how summarily the General Motors exhibit dismissed pedestrian (that is, "unimaginative") transportation. I rode with my father in wonder through the streamlined city of tomorrow, housed in a domed edifice adjacent to the Tyron and Perisphere, in the heart of Flushing Meadow. No one in this miniature industrial utopia was walking. For me, walking was "out" from then on. Any alternative was better—be it wagon, tricycle, or Irish mail (a toy handcar popular in my child-hood). Later, my friends and I would hitchhike to and from high school. The only thing more embarrassing than to be seen walking was to be caught riding in a car with your father or (God forbid!) mother.

A TALE OF TWO HOMES

Now that we are in the computer age, there is even less reason for us to walk about outside. I no longer have to go to work to use my computer; I have one at home. Our kitchen is automated, our tele-vision is interactive, and we can shop and bank on the Internet. American Express may soon shorten its admonition to "Don't leave home." My wife and I worry about how we'll manage if our machines break down.

When the Machine Stops

In "The Machine Stops," written in 1909, E. M. Forster takes the theme of don't-leave-home to its ultimate conclusion. He portrays a future society in which the people have descended to underground quar-ters—one person per hexagonal room—where their day-to-day needs and desires are met by an all-pervasive, all-accommodating automa-ton, the Machine. They venture forth from their rooms with decreas-ing frequency; there is little reason for them to do so. They can communicate with each other automatically, using transmitter, receivers, the "pneumatic post," and "blue plates" (handheld terminals in modern terms) on which the Machine projects images as well as text. Food is delivered, and waste disposed of, automatically, ad libi-tum. Medical services are delivered on demand. Music, art, literature, and science, by means of Web-like audiovisual presentations—inter-active as well as didactic—are available at the touch of a switch. And the air is always fresh.

Eventually, people have no need to leave their abodes except for the purpose of procreation. (Forster did not foresee the use of artificial insemination.) But the act of sex, no longer an act of love, is but a singular carnal responsibility to be performed with dispatch. Getting back to one's hexagonal sanctum as quickly as possible is of the high-est priority.

And there is little reason to move about, even within one's own room. An armchair and a reading desk are the only pieces of furniture. At the press of a button a hot bath rises from the floor. A bed appears on demand. (Somnolence is the only available diurnal cue, the difference between night and day having lost its meaning.) There is little reason even to move about in the chair; it takes minimal exertion to operate the buttons and switches.

As electromechanical activity replaces physical activity, flab replaces muscle. Physical powers fall into disrepute; they carry the risk of restlessness, curiosity, and (Machine forbid) rebellion. "Homelessness," banishment without respirator (the lung no longer tolerates terrestrial air) to the earth's surface and certain doom, is the penalty for independent behavior. Babies, housed in public nurseries, are sacrificed if they seem unacceptably robust at birth. There is no religion.

Whereas much of the human motor system is now vestigial, the sensory apparatus remains intact. But the reality of the world outside is perceived, from within each room, from an increasingly remote perspective. Early on, those who want to see the sights or hear the sounds of the earth's surface need only listen to a gramophone or watch a "cinematophore"—a program produced firsthand by those few who do venture, with portable respirator and "egression permit," to the surface. Eventually, however, egression is forbidden and there is no further possibility of firsthand observation. And with time the gramophones and cinematophores are transformed (Turnerized, some might say) into increasingly inexact replicas—reruns devoid of original content.

And so it is with independent thought: "Beware of firsthand ideas" is now the dictum of the day. Ideas are better acquired thirdhand than secondhand, better fourthhand than thirdhand, and so on, in a transitive relationship. Original ideas are no longer an issue; those harboring them have been banished to Homelessness.

Early on, the people responsible for the workings of the Machine understand it in its entirety. As time passes, however, division of labor prevails—"The better a man knew his own duties upon it, the less he understood the duties of his neighbor"—until there comes that crucial moment when no single person in all the world understands the Machine as a whole. This is the symbolically pivotal transition in Forster's story, for all the people in the world are now truly dependent on the Machine for life and (muscleless) limb. And with dependence comes subservience: the governing body (the Central Committee) has become a puppet; *the governed are now governed by the Machine.*

The time is now ripe for religion, and so it comes to pass. Although people still recognize intellectually that their ancestors created the Machine, they now behave as if the Machine created *them.* The word "religion" is avoided in conversation (teleconverse, if you will, conducted remotely from room to room, replete with visuals), but it is clear that the Machine is now the object of worship.

In each room, on the reading desk next to the armchair, there is one lone volume, a survivor "from the ages of litter," the *Book of the Machine.* Published by the Central Committee, this manual provides instructions for every possible use of the Machine. It is "richly bound"—new versions more so than old ones—and, increasingly, a source of spiritual comfort to those who hold it and kiss it. Technological scripture in hand, the people pray: "O Machine! O Machine!"

Diversity in worship is understood and tolerated. Some pray to the blue optic plates, others to the sound equipment, others to the Mending Apparatus, with each person imploring one or another sacred device to intercede on his or her behalf with the Machine. But there is a minimum set of tenets required of all, regardless of sect: the "Undenominational Mechanism." And there is persecution. Heretics are threatened with Homelessness.

Vashti and her son Kuno are the central figures of the story. Vashti represents the rule. A conformist, comfortable with inherited ideas, no longer capable of creative thought (and threatened and angered by those who still are), and devoid of muscle, she is philosophically at one with the Machine. Kuno, by contrast, is the exception—a renegade, independent in thought, creative in ideas, and physically active, he is philosophically wary of the Machine and continually at risk of Homelessness. As the story unfolds, Kuno calls his mother to his room (her one venture forth, done so with great reluctance) to tell her, much to her dismay, that he has climbed to the surface, up old ventilation shafts, without an egression permit and at great risk to life and limb. There he has seen life in the open air and under the sun.

For Kuno, the foray was worth the personal danger; for a brief moment in his life he was an individual, independent of the Machine. For Vashti, who wants to be spared the details of the odyssey, there is embarrassment for having mothered an ungrateful reprobate; she reproaches him angrily for breaking the rules. Kuno in turn reproves her for her unquestioning allegiance to the Machine. It goes on, back and forth. Still, during their quarrel the reader is aware of a bond, even a love, between them.

Finally, they return to their respective rooms, to visit each other no more. For the mother, life progresses peacefully; for the rebel son (we must surmise), there is increasing discontent.

Then one day, as the title of Forster's story so ominously portends, things begin to go awry. The problems are small at first but insidious—an irritating noise in a symphony from "the Brisbane school," a jarring sound emanating from an optic plate, a bit of mold on a piece of synthetic fruit (annoyances to which the people grudgingly adjust). The situation gets worse and worse, however, and with time the "stoppage" comes to interfere even with the necessities of life—a bed doesn't appear when summoned, a plate of food is inedible, and the air is no longer fresh.

People complain, but to no avail. The complaints are dutifully forwarded to the "Committee of the Mending Apparatus" (no mention of subcommittees, but we know they were there) and from there to the Central Committee, which responds with words of reassurance and a call for patience. But the situation continues to deteriorate, and at an augmented pace. The air is bad now and the lights are too dim for reading; people clutch the Book in their arms and pray in the darkness.

Then one day there is silence. The continuous, ubiquitous sound of the Machine—stimulus to every organ of Corti from the time of its embryonic inception—is gone, and the silence is terrifying. In panic, people vacate their rooms. But they cannot go far; the air is foul and the underground corridors are impassable—unlit and blocked with people struggling to move, trampling or being trampled, gasping for air or holding their breath, and dying. The Machine has stopped, and within minutes, humanity as it exists underground is extinct.

In their last few moments of life, Vashti and Kuno are reunited, and Forster offers his readers a glimmer of hope. Kuno tells his mother that when he ventured forth he saw people on the surface of the earth, living and breathing. And as the walls and ceilings collapse about them, Vashti and Kuno catch a glimpse of "untainted sky."

—◁⋙▷—

Even when Forster wrote this story in 1909, there were legitimate concerns about excessive reliance on technology in many aspects of people's lives. Still, it was the people's excessive reliance on the Machine, not the Machine itself, that led to the downfall of Forster's subterranean civilization. It can be argued that the Machine was capable of doing good, if employed with wisdom and restraint. For all the problems and ultimate horrors wrought by misuse of the Machine, Forster does say that medical services were delivered on demand. Such automated house calls, if used wisely and coupled with healthy activity, would be welcome in modern times.

In this era of high-priced medical care, technology is sometimes pointed to more as the *problem* than the solution; the machine, it is argued by well-meaning observers, is to blame for inflated costs. But in medicine as in Forster's prophetic tale, it is the misuse and overuse of the machine that is at fault, not the machine itself. If the machine helps in medical care, and as a corollary, the benefits of its use outweigh the risks, then it should be used if at all possible. If it is expensive, then we must do our best to find the funds to pay for it, while of course striving to reduce the costs.

Fortunately, most good machines in medicine have become less and less expensive with more and more use; the autoanalyzer, the CAT scan, the MRI machine, and the computer itself come quickly to mind. Furthermore, judicious use of these machines is for the most part *less* expensive (as well as medically better) than are the older methods the machines have replaced. Forster's underground people misused and overused their Machine, just as now some clinicians misuse and overuse machines to the detriment of their patients and the finances of medicine. But when used wisely and well, the machine in medicine, and in particular the computer, in keeping with the theme of *Cybermedicine,* is a *solution* and not a problem.

Let me turn then to an example of the computer as a solution in health care in the home.

When the Home Is Also the Clinic: The Tale of One Real Child

Whether medical care is primarily the responsibility of the doctor or the patient is often dictated by supply and demand. If the biochemistry of insulin or the physiology of the pancreas were such that a child with diabetes needed only one injection of insulin per year, it is likely that the diabetes expert in the academic medical center would administer the insulin—at the hospital and at considerable expense. If the child needed an injection every six months, the pediatrician would do it in the office; if every three months, the nurse practitioner. But the need is typically twice a day, and it is the parent or older child who gives the injection at home, with skill and without professional assistance. There is no other way.

On the other hand, the family needs guidance. When their clinical interactions occur in a doctor's office rather than their home, the doctor rarely sees their living situation. But this is where they will try to carry out the plans they have made in dialogue with the doctor. In other words, there may be a disparity between plans made in the controlled environment of a physician's examining room and the realities of life in the patient's home. My family and I have experienced this problem firsthand, and the interactive computer has been of great help to us at home.

Five years ago, our daughter and her husband noticed that their seventeen-month-old toddler, our grandson Sean, had been drinking a lot of water for several days and urinating heavily since the evening before; his diaper was soaked in the morning. Sean was alert and active, but Alison and Chris were concerned, observing parents as they are. They took Sean to the pediatrician. A urine test was positive for glucose. When they telephoned my wife and me, Alison and Chris were taking Sean (and their three-year-old, James) to the university hospital in the city for definitive diagnosis.

During Sean's brief stay in the hospital he was given excellent medical care. Insulin was administered, and Sean's blood glucose level and fluid and electrolyte imbalance were brought quickly under control. The doctors and nurses did their best to be pleasant. But there were problems with communication. Alison and Chris were given the instant short course on juvenile diabetes: doctors, doctors in training, nurses, nurses in training, nutritionists, nutritionists in training, and various auxiliary health care workers traipsed in and out of the little boy's room, each offering interpretations and advice from a new perspective. The upshot was a conflicting array of directives and advice: "Sean doesn't have to eat everything on the tray." "It's imperative that Sean eat everything on the tray." "You can always get in touch with the doctor when you need help." "We mustn't bother the doctor now." "Give him his insulin and wait a half hour before you feed him." "You don't have to wait before feeding him."

The importance of diet was emphasized, and in this case everyone agreed. Sean was to receive three meals a day, each containing forty-two grams of carbohydrate in roughly equal amounts of starch, dairy food, and fruit, with three snacks between meals (seven grams of carbohydrate in the morning, seven grams in the afternoon, and fifteen grams before bedtime). For Sean's first breakfast in the hospital, Alison and Chris dutifully ordered three-fourths of a cup of Cheerios (fifteen grams of carbohydrate), one cup of whole milk (twelve grams), and half a cup of orange juice (fifteen grams). A tray appeared with a bowl of grits, a glass of skim milk, two sausages, and a cup of black coffee.

I don't mean to imply that there was no effort at good communication. The house officers were helpful and sympathetic. The nurses were readily available day and night, doing their best to accommodate the patients and their families (there were many seriously ill children and concerned parents on the pediatric service). The nurses' instructions on using the glucometer and administering insulin were given with skill and patience. Alison and Chris learned quickly how to prick a finger, put a drop of blood on the strip, read the blood glucose determination, measure the insulin in a syringe, and give Sean the injection. A great many pamphlets and booklets appeared, some making sense and some not. Most of the reading material had been developed for older children; seventeen months is very young for the onset of diabetes.

Sean was discharged on the dietary program begun in the hospital (without the coffee) and a "sliding scale" formula for insulin. The senior physicians had made it clear that the goal was to keep his blood glucose between 100 and 200, difficult as this would be. They had *not* made it clear that this was an ideal goal; that meeting it consistently would be *impossible*. In addition, they had not explained that tight control of glucose levels would be much more important after puberty than before.

In young children with diabetes, if either end of the glucose spectrum, particularly the low end, can be avoided, this is good management. If the blood level can be kept between 100 and 200 half the time, that is about the best one can hope for. And even with the best-laid plans and under the best of circumstances, there will be wide, anxiety-provoking fluctuations between hyperglycemia and hypoglycemia. Parents must learn to live with this.

The first month at home was the hardest. But somehow the family got through it, with the help of relatives and friends. (Soon there was a new baby, Catherine.) The senior doctor's offer—"You can call us any time"—proved accurate; Alison and Chris *could* call them any time. But most of the time they were told to wait for a return phone call, and sometimes it never came.

On the first Saturday at home Sean was vomiting and took little by mouth. The doctor on call recommended altering the insulin dosage, giving Sean whatever he would take by mouth, and most important, giving him fluids if he could hold them down, to prevent dehydration. Sean was better on Sunday, but Monday morning he started vomiting again. This time the senior pediatric diabetologist came to the phone (his secretary cajoled him upon Alison's insistence). He proceeded to scold Alison for doing what his colleague had recommended two days before. Later that day, Alison and Chris took Sean back to the hospital for rehydration. Fortunately, the resident who had been their favorite doctor during the earlier hospitalization was on hand. She offered advice and comfort, and stayed by the bedside to supervise the administration of the intravenous fluids. Sean was back home in a few hours, much improved.

THE GLUCOMETER. During his first year with diabetes, Sean's insulin schedule was determined by his glucometer readings. Every morning he got 2 units of long-acting insulin. This was combined with 1 unit of regular insulin if his glucose was 70 to 100 mg per deciliter, 1.5 units if his glucose was 101 to 150, 2 units if it was 151 to 200, 2.5 units if 201 to 300, and 3 units if over 300. In the evening he got 1 unit of long-acting insulin together with 0.5 unit of regular insulin if the glucose was 101 to 150, 1 unit if 151 to 200, 1.5 units if 201 to 300, and 2 units if over 300.

The glucometer is a wonderful machine, a specialized handheld computer made available for home use some eighteen years ago. It boggles my mind to think of the management of diabetes before the glucometer was developed, when families had to rely on the presence or absence of glucose in the urine. There was a lot of guessing. If the urine was free of glucose, this could be good (normoglycemia) or bad (hypoglycemia). Insulin dosages were determined by the urinary glucose level, and with toddlers like Sean, the renal threshold for glucose can be quite variable. The traditional intermittent visit to the clinic for a venipuncture was more symbolic than practical; a single, random glucose value is hardly indicative of day-to-day control.

With the glucometer, Sean's blood glucose could be measured many times a day, before his insulin injection, before each meal, and whenever there was cause for worry—when he had an upper respiratory tract infection, for example—although his parents didn't want to prick those little fingers more often than they had to. (Sean was too young to tell them how he felt; they were greatly relieved when a year later he first said, "I feel shaky.") His first glucometer required a large drop of blood, which was not always easy to elicit from a diminutive digit. Alison or Chris would put a warm compress on one of Sean's fingers to make a usable drop more likely. But sometimes they would have to prick a second finger, sometimes a third or fourth. Another parent (rather than a doctor) told Alison about the Glucometer Elite, a new computer that worked with a small droplet of blood. This made life much easier for Sean and his parents, who from then on rarely had to prick a finger a second time. Alison then passed this information on to other parents in her Juvenile Diabetes Foundation chat group on the Internet. (There is active research now being done on a noninvasive glucometer, which will be a godsend for insulin-dependent diabetics.)

Approaching the "terrible twos," Sean was beginning to assert his independence, and "no" had a prominent place in his vocabulary. He was particularly apt to use this word at mealtimes, which have special importance in the life of a diabetic child. It was imperative for Sean to eat after his insulin injection. His breakfast and dinner were to be eaten, in theory, after thirty minutes. I am saying "in theory" advisedly. On one hand, there is the ideal, harmonious relationship between toddler and parent, with the calm, smiling parent measuring a blood glucose level of precisely 151 mg per deciliter, administering 4 units of insulin, and after thirty minutes, feeding forty-two grams of carbohydrate. This was the picture dictated by the staff of the academic division of pediatric diabetology. On the other hand, there is the reality of a little boy in his high chair in the dining room, lips tight, masseters fully contracted (mouth opening only for as long as it takes to say "No!" to an approaching spoon)—the anxious interplay between an uncomprehending two-year-old and a parent faced with the prospect of insulin shock.

THE PROBLEM. It's 7:30 in the morning. You and your little boy have the daily diabetes ordeal ahead of you. You place the equipment within easy reach and sit in a straight-backed chair. You call your child, who runs over and gives your leg a hug. You put him in your lap. You look at your notebook to check which finger to use. You swab the finger with alcohol, press the pricking device against it, distract your child with some gentle words, and press the button. He barely flinches; the spring action is well designed and the small lancet is very sharp. You touch his finger to the glucometer strip. He reaches for the pricking device. You quickly remove the lancet and let him grab the device, which he examines eagerly. Now *he's* in control. After thirty seconds, he says "beep." After forty-five seconds, the glucometer says "beep." You look at the reading anxiously—220. You relax.

The little guy hops down and runs about happily. You draw the insulin into the small syringe—2 units long-acting, 2.5 units regular. This is tricky; the amounts are small and exact measurement is impossible. You just want to be as close as possible. You check your notebook again—"right thigh." You call him again. He comes, but a little more slowly this time. He's up on your lap; you swab a place on his thigh, gently create a fold of skin, talk diversion-type talk, and inject the insulin. He whimpers briefly. You give him a hug. He gives you a hug. Breakfast in thirty minutes.

The little guy is now in his high chair. On the tray is a small bowl of Cheerios (fifteen grams of carbohydrate), carefully measured. "It's time for breakfast," you say with a smile, "You like Cheerios, don't you?" You look away for a moment and hear a forceful "No!" from the high chair. You turn back. The cereal is on the floor. You begin to worry; the insulin is working and he needs to eat. You hand him his "Barney" cup—orange juice (fifteen grams), carefully measured. You turn to your other children for a moment. Bang, splash. You turn back. There's a big grin on the boy's face; he has tested the law of gravity and it holds. You move quickly to the kitchen, peel a banana—five inches (fifteen grams)—and hand it to him. He does his Pedro Martinez windup. You retrieve the banana in the nick of time. You give him a small piece of it, which he eats. You relax a little. His appetite has prevailed. He eats his new serving of Cheerios, carefully measured. You relax a bit more. He drinks his milk. You are feeling better.

Two hours pass. It's time for his snack. He drinks his milk, a quarter of a cup (three grams), carefully measured. You give him a peanut cracker (four grams). He scurries off. Minutes later he returns empty-handed. Oh God! Did he eat it or drop it behind the couch? Should you check his blood glucose again? You decide to give him another cracker (too much is better than too little). He eats the cracker under your watchful eye and is off to play. In two hours it will be time for lunch.

A SOLUTION. Finding a good doctor is, of course, most important, and the family was particularly fortunate to find Barry Reiner, a knowledgeable, compassionate, supportive, and readily available physician, who worked with Alison and Chris as peers, on behalf of Sean. When Sean was five, Alison, Chris, and Barry replaced Sean's insulin injections with an insulin pump, another marvelous, pager-sized computer that injects insulin, in preprogrammed and, at mealtimes, manually designated amounts, through a catheter implanted just beneath the skin. Although one of the youngest children to have a pump—and there have been problems to be worked out, such as when the catheter becomes kinked or dislodged—Sean loves his pump, and it has made life substantially easier for Alison and Chris. (Once a pump is developed that can monitor subcutaneous glucose levels continuously—and we eagerly await this—Sean and other diabetics will have the equivalent of an artificial pancreas, a computer that can provide insulin continually, as needed.)

Cybermedicine can also help. With the thriving technology of tele-converse, patients and parents of patients with access to the Internet can communicate with their doctors and with other patients and parents. (My dream, of course, is that access will become universal in the near future.) And Alison and Chris are regular users of e-mail, newsgroups, mailing lists, and chat groups (Sean, at six, is learning). In communication with others who share the problems associated with diabetes, they have received companionship and reassurance as well as practical suggestions. And they in turn have been of great help to others.

In the future, cybermedicine programs will be available on the Internet that simulate the time-honored, one-on-one conversation between patient and doctor, with the collective wisdom of many doctors and in a convenient place for the family. This will, I believe, be of great assistance to families during the intervals between appointments with their physicians and will serve to enhance communication between family members and physicians at the time of their visits.

Despite the difficulties I have described, Sean and his family are doing very well. He is a brilliant, loving, beautiful little boy, if you will permit a grandfather's assessment.

CONCLUSION

I look forward to the time when doctors will leave their cloistered clinical environments, literally as well as by computer-based telecommunication, to familiarize themselves with the home environments of their patients, and thereby close the gap between prescription and implementation. For the pediatric diabetologist, an even more informative experience would be to raise a diabetic child. But short of this, firsthand knowledge of the day-to-day life of the patient and the patient's family could go a long way.

I am in complete agreement with Forster's admonition—all the more remarkable in that it was written in 1909—that abdication to a machine would lead to disaster. But Forster was not opposed to machines themselves; he appreciated the societal benefits of technology. He was opposed, as I am, to the loss of human control over machines. And we must guard against this with computers in medicine.

Whereas it is not necessary for users to understand the inner workings of computers, it is of the utmost importance for developers to understand the systems they develop, to recognize that they are responsible for their systems and accountable to their users, and to make sure their bond of trust with their users is never broken.

For the user, the off button should always be placed in a prominent location. And of course we should all get plenty of fresh air and exercise.

—◦◦◦—

One day, not long ago, I was late for a meeting. Self-absorbed and a bit irritable, I rushed to the stairs, ready to descend in haste. Shortly thereafter, I wrote this little poem:

ENCOUNTER ON THE STAIRS

Next to Children's Hospital, in a hurry
Down the stairs, two at a time
Slowed down by a family, moving slowly
Blocking the stairway, I'm in a hurry
I stop, annoyed, I'm in a hurry
Seeing me, they move to the side
A woman says softly, "sorry" in Spanish
I look down in passing, there's a little boy
Unsteady in gait, holding onto an arm
Head shaved, stitches in scalp, patch over eye, thin and pale
He catches my eye and gives me a smile
My walk is slower for the rest of the day.

—⁓—

When use of the computer in medicine liberates us from bureaucratic drudgery, we can of course let our schedules be filled with yet additional administrative chores. But we clinicians do have another choice. We can use this computer-enabled freedom to stay the ever-accelerating pace of our lives, to reflect more carefully on what really matters, and to spend more time with our patients. Perhaps we can walk more slowly for the rest of our days.

ᵐᵐ Bibliography and Further Reading

New Preface

Davis, J. B. (ed.). *Health and Medicine on the Internet: Annual Guide to the World Wide Web (Consumer Edition).* Los Angeles: Health Information Press, 1997.

Davis, J. B. (ed.). *Health and Medicine on the Internet: Annual Guide to the World Wide Web for Healthcare Professionals.* Los Angeles: Practice Management Information Corporation, 1997.

Eder, L. *Managing Healthcare Information Systems with Web-Enabled Technologies.* Hershey, Pa.: Idea Group, 2000.

Eng, T. R., and Gustafson, D. H. (eds.). *Wired for Health and Well-Being: The Emergence of Interactive Health Communication.* Washington, D.C.: Office of Disease Prevention and Health Promotion: U.S. Department of Health and Human Services, 1999.

Ferguson, T. *Health On-line: How to Find Health Information, Support Groups, and Self-Help Communities in Cyberspace.* Reading, Mass.: Addison-Wesley, 1996.

Ferguson, T. *The Ferguson Report.* Available on-line: http://www.ferguson-report.com.

Gibbs, S. R., Sullivan-Fowler, M., and Rowe, N. W. (eds.). *A Guide to Exploring the Internet and Discovering the Top Health Care Resources.* St. Louis, Mo.: Mosby, 1996.

Jacquez, J. A. (ed.). *Computer Diagnosis and Diagnostic Methods: The Proceedings of the Second Conference on the Diagnostic Process Held at the University of Michigan.* Springfield, Ill.: Thomas, 1972.

Louis Harris & Associates. "Sixty Million Seek Health Info On-line in the US." *Nua Internet Surveys 1999.* Available on-line: http://www.nua.ie/surveys.

Maxwell, B. *How to Find Health Information on the Internet.* Washington, D.C.: Congressional Quarterly Inc., 1998.

Nua. "Cyber Dialogue: Doctors Keep Work Offline." *Nua Internet Surveys 2001.* Available on-line: http://www.nua.ie/surveys.

Ryer, J. C. *HealthNet: Your Essential Resource for the Most Up-to-Date Medical Information Online.* New York: Wiley, 1997.

Schneider, J. S., and Lidsky, T. I. *The Doctor's Always In: A Guide to 1,100+ Best Health and Medical Information Sites on the Internet.* Cherry Hill, N.J.: NeuroInformatics, 1998.

Sharp, V. F., and Sharp, R. M. *Web Doctor: Finding the Best Care Online.* New York: St. Martin's Griffin, 1998.

Shortliffe, E. H., and Perreault, L. E. (eds.) with Wiederhold, G., and Fagan, L. M. (assoc. eds.). *Medical Informatics: Computer Applications in Health Care and Biomedicine.* New York: Springer-Verlag, 2000.

Weiner, N. *Cybernetics.* New York: Wiley, 1961.

Preface to First Edition

Collen, M. F. *A History of Medical Informatics in the United States, 1950 to 1990.* Bethesda, Md.: American Medical Informatics Association, 1995.

McCarty, R. J., Kanter, T., and Sopanen, J. *Lifeline.* Videotape documentary of cybermedicine systems developed for Boston's Beth Israel and Brigham and Women's hospitals by the Center for Clinical Computing. Produced by RJM Associates, 1995.

McCarty, R. J., Kanter, T., and Sopanen, J. Video archives of interviews of users and developers of cybermedicine systems in Beth Israel and Brigham and Women's hospitals. Produced by RJM Associates, 1995.

Rogers, C. R. *Client-Centered Therapy.* Boston: Houghton Mifflin, 1965.

Shaw, G. B. *Man and Superman: A Comedy and Philosophy.* Baltimore: Penguin, 1952. (Originally published 1903.)

Slack, W. V. "Patient Power." In J. A. Jacquez (ed.), *Computer Diagnosis and Diagnostic Methods: The Proceedings of the Second Conference on the Diagnostic Process Held at the University of Michigan.* Springfield, Ill.: Thomas, 1972.

Slack, W. V. "The Patient's Right to Decide." *Lancet,* 1977, *2,* 240.

Chapter One (Providing Information to Patients)

Alcoholics Anonymous. New York: Alcoholics Anonymous Publishing, 1955.

Haggard, H. W. *Devils, Drugs, and Doctors.* Boston: Charles River Books, 1980.

Machiavelli, N. *The Prince.* (G. Bull, trans.). Hammondsport, England: Penguin Books, 1981. (Originally published 1513.)

Slack, W. V. "Patient Counseling by Computer." In S. Zoog and S. Yarnall (eds.), *The Changing Health Care Team*. Seattle: Medical Communications and Services Association, 1976.

Slack, W. V. "Compugraphy." *M.D. Computing*, 1991, *8*(6), 342–346.

Slack, W. V. "When the Home Is Also the Clinic." *M.D. Computing*, 1996, *13*(6), 465–468.

Spock, B. *Dr. Spock's Baby and Child Care: Sixth Edition Fully Revised and Updated for the 1990s.* New York: NAL/Dutton, 1992.

Chapter Two (Patient-Computer Dialogue)

Baer, L., Brown-Beasley, M. W., Sorce, J., and Henriques, A. I. "Computer-Assisted Telephone Administration of a Structured Interview for Obsessive-Compulsive Disorder." *American Journal of Psychiatry,* 1993, *150*(11), 1737–1738.

Bana, D. S., Leviton, A., Swidler, C., Slack, W. V., and Graham, J. R. "A Computer-Based Headache Interview: Acceptance by Patients and Physicians." *Headache,* 1980, *20*, 85–89.

Bennett, S. E., Lawrence, R. S., Fleischmann, K. H., Gifford, C. S., and Slack, W. V. "Profile of Women Practicing Breast Self-Examination." *Journal of the American Medical Association,* 1983, *249*(4), 488–491.

Bergeron, B., and Locke, S. E. "Speech Recognition as a User Interface." *M.D. Computing,* 1990, *6*(1), 329–334.

Berne, E. *Transactional Analysis in Psychotherapy.* New York: Grove Press, 1961.

Bleich, H. L. "The Kaiser Permanente Health Plan, Dr. Morris F. Collen, and Automated Multiphasic Testing." *M.D. Computing,* 1994, *11*(3), 136–139.

Bleich, H. L. "Wesley A. Clark, Charles E. Molnar, and the LINC." *M.D. Computing,* 1994, *11*(5), 269–270.

Bock, B., Niaura, R., Fontes, A., and Bock, F. "Acceptability of Computer Assessments Among Ethnically Diverse, Low-Income Smokers." *American Journal of Health Promotion,* 1999, *13*, 299–304.

Brodman, K., Erdmann, A. J., Jr., Lorge, I., and Wolff, H. G. "Cornell Medical Index: Adjunct to Medical Interview." *Journal of the American Medical Association,* 1949, *140*, 530–534.

Brodman, K., Van Woerkom, A. J., Erdmann, A. J., Jr., and Goldstein, L. S. "Interpretation of Symptoms with a Data-Processing Machine." *Archives of Internal Medicine,* 1959, *103*, 776–782.

Chun, R.W.M., Van Cura, L. J., Spencer, M., and Slack, W. V. "Computer Interviewing of Patients with Epilepsy." *Epilepsy,* 1976, *17*, 371–375.

Clark, W. A., and Molnar, C. E. "A Description of the LINC." In R. W. Stacy and B. D. Waxman (eds.), *Computers in Biomedical Research*. Vol. 2. New York: Academic Press, 1965.

Collen, M. F., Rubin, L., Neyman, J., Dantzig, G. B., Baer, R. M., and Siegelaub, A. B. "Automated Multiphasic Screening and Diagnosis." *American Journal of Public Health*, 1964, *54*, 741–750.

Coombs, G. J., Murray, W. R., and Krahn, D. W. "Automated Medical Histories: Factors Determining Patient Performance." *Computers and Biomedical Research*, 1970, *3*, 178–181.

Erdman, H. P., Klein, M. H., and Greist, J. H. "Direct Patient Computer Interviewing." *Journal of Consulting and Clinical Psychology*, 1985, *53*, 760–773.

Evans, S., and Gormican, A. "The Computer in Retrieving Dietary History Data." *Journal of the American Dietetic Association*, 1973, *63*, 397–407.

Fulton, S. M. "Speak Softly, Carry a Big Chip: Using Speech Recognition Software Takes Patience and Computer Power." *New York Times*, Mar. 30, 2000. Available on-line: http://www.out-loud.com.

Gottlieb, G. L., Beers, R. F., Bernecker, C., and Samter, M. "An Approach to Automation of Medical Interviews." *Computers and Biomedical Research*, 1972, *5*, 99–107.

Greist, J. H., and Slack, W. V. "A Computer-Conducted Interview for Intern Applicants." *Journal of Medical Education*, 1970, *45*, 941–944.

Greist, J. H., Van Cura, L. J., and Kneppreth N. P. "A Computer Interview for Emergency Room Patients. *Computers and Biomedical Research*, 1973, *6*, 257–265.

Grossman, J. H., Barnett, G. O., McGuire, M. T., and Swedlow, D. B. "Evaluation of Computer-Acquired Patient Histories." *Journal of the American Medical Association*, 1971, *215*(8), 1286–1291.

Hasley, S. "A Comparison of Computer-Based Personal Interviews for the Gynecologic History Update." *Obstetrics and Gynecology*, 1995, *84*(4), 494–498.

Haug, P. J., Warner, H. R., Clayton, P. D., Schmidt, C. D., Pearl, J. E., Farney, R. J., Crapo, R. O., Tocino, I., Morrison, W. J., and Frederick, P. R. "A Decision-Driven System to Collect the Patient History." *Computers and Biomedical Research*, 1987, *20*, 193–207.

Hicks, G. P., Gieschen, M. M., Slack, W. V., and Larson, F. C. "Routine Use of a Small Digital Computer in the Clinical Laboratory." *Journal of the American Medical Association*, 1966, *196*, 973–978.

Houziaux, M. O., and Lefebve, P. J. "Historical and Methodological Aspects of Computer-Assisted Medical History Taking." *Medical Informatics (London)*, 1986, *11*, 129–143.

Jacquez, J. A. (ed.). *Computer Diagnosis and Diagnostic Methods: The Proceedings of the Second Conference on the Diagnostic Process Held at the University of Michigan*. Springfield, Ill.: Thomas, 1972.

Kafka, F. *The Castle. A New Translation Based on the Restored Text.* (M. Harman, trans.). New York: Schocken, 1998. (Originally published 1926.)

Koestler, A. *Darkness at Noon.* (D. Hardy, trans.). New York: Macmillan, 1987. (Originally published 1941.)

Kohlmeier, L., Mendez, M., McDuffie, J., and Miller, M. "Computer-Assisted Self-Interviewing: A Multimedia Approach to Dietary Assessment." *American Journal of Clinical Nutrition*, 1997, *65*(4 Supplement), 1275S–1281S.

Lessler, J. T., and O'Reilly, J. M. "Mode of Interview and Reporting of Sensitive Issues: Design and Implementation of Audio Computer-Assisted Self-Interviewing." In *NIDA Research Monograph*. Research Triangle Institute, N.C., 1997.

Leviton, A., Slack, W. V., Bana, D., and Graham, J. R. "Age-Related Headache Characteristics." *Archives of Neurology*, 1984, *41*, 762–764.

Leviton, A., Slack, W. V., Masek, B., Bana, D., and Graham, J. R. "A Computerized Behavioral Assessment for Children with Headaches." *Headache*, 1984, *24*, 182–185.

Linberg, G., Seensalu, R., Nilsson, L. H., Forsell, P., Kagar, L., and Knill-Jones, R. P. "Transferability of a Computer System for Medical History Taking and Decision Support in Dyspepsia: A Comparison of Indicants for Peptic Ulcer Disease." *Scandinavian Journal of Gastroenterology Supplement*, 1987, *128*, 190–196.

Lutner, R. E., Roizen, M. F., Stocking, C. B., Thisted, R. A., Kim, S., Duke, P. C., Pompei, P., and Kassel, C. K. "The Automated Interview Versus the Personal Interview: Do Patient Responses to Preoperative Health Questions Differ?" *Anesthesiology*, 1991, *75*(3), 394–400.

Marvel, M. K., Epstein, R. M., Flowers, K., and Beckman, H. B. "Soliciting the Patient's Agenda: Have We Improved?" *Journal of the American Medical Association*, 1999, *281*, 283–287.

Mayne, J. G., Weksel, W., and Sholtz, P. N. "Toward Automating the Medical History." *Mayo Clinic Proceedings*, 1968, *43*, 1–25.

Metzger, D. S., Koblin, B., Turner, C., Navaline, H., Valenti, F., Holte, S., Gross, M., Sheon, A., Miller, H., Cooley, P., and Seage, G. R., III. "Randomized Controlled Trial of Audio Computer-Assisted Self-Interviewing: Utility and Acceptability in Longitudinal Studies. HIVNET Vaccine Preparedness Study Protocol Team." *American Journal of Epidemiology*, 2000, *152*, 99–106.

Millstein, S. G., and Irwin, C. E., Jr. "Acceptability of Computer-Acquired Sexual Histories in Adolescent Girls." *Journal of Pediatrics*, 1983, *103*, 815–819.

Paperny, D. M., and Hedberg, V. A. "Computer-Assisted Health Counselor Visits: A Low-Cost Model for Comprehensive Adolescent Preventive Services." *Archives of Pediatric Adolescent Medicine*, 1999, *153*, 63–67.

Pauker, S. G., Gorry, G. A., Kassirer, J. P., and Schwartz, W. B. "Towards the Simulation of Clinical Cognition: Taking a Present Illness by Computer." *American Journal of Medicine*, 1976, *60*, 981–996.

Peckham, B. M., Slack, W. V., Carr, W. F., Van Cura, L. J., and Schultz, A. E. "Computerized Data Collection in the Management of Uterine Cancer." *Clinical Obstetrics and Gynecology*, 1967, *10*, 1003–1015.

Pierce, B. "The Use of Instant Medical History in a Rural Clinic. Case Study of the Use of Computers in an Arkansas Physician's Office." *Journal of the Arkansas Medical Society*, 2000, *96*, 444–447.

Porter, S. C., Silvia, M. T., Fleisher, G. R., Kohane, I. S., Homer, C. J., and Mandl, K. D. "Parents as Direct Contributors to the Medical Record: Validation of Their Electronic Input." *Annals of Emergency Medicine*, 2000, *35*, 346–352.

Pringle, M. "Using Computers to Take Patient Histories." *British Medical Journal*, 1988, *297*, 697–698.

Quaak, M. J., Westerman, R. F., Schout, J. A., Hasman, A., and van Bemmel, J. H. "Patient Appreciations of Computerized Medical Interviews." *Medical Informatics (London)*, 1986, *11*, 339–350.

Savage, L. J. "Diagnosis and the Bayesian Viewpoint." In J. A. Jacquez (ed.), *Computer Diagnosis and Diagnostic Methods: The Proceedings of the Second Conference on the Diagnostic Process Held at the University of Michigan.* Springfield, Ill.: Thomas, 1972.

Skinner, H. A., Allen B. A., McIntosh, M. C., and Palmer, W. H. "Lifestyle Assessment: Applying Microcomputers in Family Practice." *British Medical Journal (Clinical Research Edition)*, 1985, *290*, 212–214.

Slack, W. "Computer-Based Interviewing System Dealing with Nonverbal Behavior As Well As Keyboard Responses." *Science*, 1971, *171*, 84–87.

Slack, W. V. "Patient Power." In J. A. Jacquez (ed.), *Computer Diagnosis and*

Diagnostic Methods: The Proceedings of the Second Conference on the Diagnostic Process Held at the University of Michigan. Springfield, Ill.: Thomas, 1972.

Slack, W. V. "The Patient's Right to Decide." *Lancet,* 1977, *2,* 240.

Slack, W. V. "A History of Computerized Medical Interviews." *M.D. Computing,* 1984, *1*(5), 52–59, 68.

Slack, W. V. "Measurement of Intelligence: Misplaced Trust and the Lure of Prophecy." *M.D. Computing,* 1995, *12*(5), 363–372.

Slack, W. V. "Brave New Interviewer." *Harvard Medical Alumni Bulletin,* 1996, *69*(4), 44–49.

Slack, W. V. "Cybermedicine: How Computing Empowers Patients for Better Health Care." In B. Cesnik, A. T. McCray, and J. R. Scherrer (eds.), *MEDINFO '98.* Amsterdam: IOS Press, 1998.

Slack, W. V. "Patient-Computer Dialogue: A Review." In J. H. van Bemmel and A. T. McCray (eds.), *Yearbook of Medical Informatics 2000: Patient-centered Systems.* Stuttgart, Germany: Schattauer, 2000.

Slack, W. V., Hicks, G. P., Reed, C. E., and Van Cura, L. J. "A Computer-Based Medical History System." *New England Journal of Medicine,* 1966, *274*(4), 194–198.

Slack, W. V., Leviton, A., Bennett, S. E., Fleischmann, K. H., and Lawrence, R. S. "Relation Between Age, Education, and Time to Respond to Questions in a Computer-Based Medical Interview." *Computers and Biomedical Research,* 1988, *21,* 78–84.

Slack, W. V., and Van Cura, L. J. "Computer-Based Patient Interviewing. Parts I & II." *Postgraduate Medicine,* 1968, *43,* 68–74, 115–120.

Slack, W. V., and Van Cura, L. J. "Patient Reaction to Computer-Based Medical Interviewing." *Computers and Biomedical Research,* 1968, *1,* 527–531.

Stead, W. W., Hammond, W. E., and Estes, E. H. "Evaluation of an Audio Mode of the Automated Medical History." *Methods of Information in Medicine,* 1977, *16,* 20–23.

Stead, W. W., Heyman, A., Thompson, H. K., and Hammond, W. E. "Computer-Assisted Interview of Patients with Functional Headaches." *Archives of Internal Medicine,* 1972, *129,* 1–12.

Turner, C. F., Ku, L., Rogers, S. M., Lindberg, L. D., Pleck, J. H., and Sonenstein, F. L. "Adolescent Sexual Behavior, Drug Use, and Violence: Increased Reporting with Computer Survey Technology." *Science,* 1998, *280*(5365), 867–873.

Underhill, L. H., and Slack, W. V. "Computerized Histories Have Many Functions." *Computer News for Physicians,* 1987, *5,* 8–9.

Van Cura, L. J., Jensen, N. M., Greist, J. H., Lewis, W. R., and Frey, S. R. "Venereal Disease: Interviewing and Teaching by Computer." *American Journal of Public Health,* 1975, *65,* 1159–1164.

Wald, J. S., Rind, D., Safran, C., Kowaloff, H., Barker, R., and Slack, W. V. "Patient Entries in the Electronic Medical Record: An Interactive Interview Used in Primary Care." In R. M. Gardner (ed.), *American Medical Informatics Association: The Proceedings of the Nineteenth Annual Symposium on Computer Applications in Medical Care.* Philadelphia: Hanley & Belfus, 1995.

Warner, H. R., Rutherford, B. D., and Houtchens, B. A. "A Sequential Bayesian Approach to History Taking and Diagnosis." *Computers and Biomedical Research,* 1972, *5,* 256–262.

Chapter Three (Cybermedicine as a Patient's Assistant)

Angle, H. V., Johnson, T., Grebenkemper, N. S., and Ellinwood, E. H. "Computer Interview Support of Clinicians." *Professional Psychology,* Feb. 1979, pp. 49–57.

Barry, M. J., Fowler, F. J., Jr., Mulley, A. G., Jr., Henderson, J. V., Jr., and Wennberg, J. E. "Patient Reaction to a Program Designed to Facilitate Patient Participation in Treatment Decisions for Benign Prostatic Hyperplasia." *Medical Care,* 1995, *33*(8), 771–782.

Bleich, H. L., Beckley, R. F., Horowitz, G., Jackson, J., Moody, E., Franklin, C., Goodman, S. R., McKay, M. W., Pope, R. A., Walden, T., Bloom, S. A., and Slack, W. V. "Clinical Computing in a Teaching Hospital." *New England Journal of Medicine,* 1985, *312*(12), 756–764.

Bloom, S., White, R., Beckley, R., and Slack, W. "Converse: A Means to Write, Edit, Administer and Summarize Computer-Based Dialogue." *Computers and Biomedical Research,* 1978, *11,* 167–175.

Brennan, P. F., Ripich, S., and Moore, S. M. "The Use of Home-Based Computers to Support Persons Living with AIDS/ARC." *Journal of Community Health Nursing,* 1991, *8*(1), 3–14.

Deyo, R. A., Cherkin, D. C., Weinstein, J., Howe, J., Ciol, M., and Mulley, A. G., Jr. "Involving Patients in Clinical Decisions: Impact of an Interactive Video Program on Use of Back Surgery." *Medical Care,* 2000, *38,* 959–969.

Fisher, L. A., Johnson, T. S., Porter, D., Bleich, H. L., and Slack, W. V. "Collection of a Clean Voided Urine Specimen: A Comparison Among Spoken, Written, and Computer-Based Instructions." *American Journal of Public Health,* 1977, *67,* 640–644.

Flatley-Brennan, P. "Computer Network Home Care Demonstration:

A Randomized Trial in Persons Living with AIDS." *Computers in Biology and Medicine,* 1998, *28,* 489–508.

Gustafson, D. H., Bosworth, K., Hawkins, R. P., Boberg, E. W., and Bricker, E. "CHESS: A Computer-Based System for Providing Information, Referrals, Decision Support and Social Support to People Facing Medical and Other Health-Related Crises." In M. E. Frisse (ed.), *Proceedings of the Sixteenth Annual Symposium on Computer Applications in Medical Care.* Baltimore: American Medical Informatics Association, 1992.

Gustafson, D. H., Hawkins, R., Boberg, E., Pingree, S., Serlin, R. E., Graziano, F., and Chan, C. L. "Impact of a Patient-Centered, Computer-Based Health Information/Support System." *American Journal of Preventive Medicine,* 1999, *16,* 1–9.

Lieberman, J. A., III. "Compliance Issues in Primary Care." *Journal of Clinical Psychiatry Supplement,* 1996, *57*(7), 76–82.

Mulley, A. G. "Supporting the Patient's Role in Decision Making." *Journal of Occupational Medicine,* 1990, *32*(12), 1227–1228.

Shaw, B. R., McTavish, F., Hawkins, R., Gustafson, D. H., and Pingree, S. "Experiences of Women with Breast Cancer: Exchanging Social Support Over the CHESS Computer Network." *Journal of Health Community,* 2000, *5,* 135–159.

Slack, W. V. "Patient Counseling by Computer." In S. Zoog and S. Yarnall (eds.), *The Changing Health Care Team.* Seattle: Medical Communications and Services Association, 1976.

Slack, W. V. "The Patient's Right to Decide." *Lancet,* 1977, *2,* 240.

Slack, W. V. "Cybermedicine: How Computing Empowers Patients for Better Health Care." In B. Cesnik, A. T. McCray, and J. R. Scherrer (eds.), *MEDINFO '98.* Amsterdam: IOS Press, 1998.

Slack, W. V. "Patient-Computer Dialogue: A Review." In J. H. van Bemmel and A. T. McCray (eds.), *Yearbook of Medical Informatics 2000: Patient-centered Systems.* Stuttgart, Germany: Schattauer, 2000.

Slack, W., Porter, D., Witschi, J., Sullivan, M., Buxbaum, R., and Stare, F. "Dietary Interviewing by Computer: An Experimental Approach to Counseling." *Journal of the American Dietetic Association,* 1976, *69,* 514–517.

Slack, W. V., Safran, C., Kowaloff, H. B., Pearce, J., and Delbanco, T. L. "A Computer-Administered Health Screening Interview for Hospital Personnel." *M.D. Computing,* 1995, *12*(1), 25–30.

Stamm, W. E. "Urinary Tract Infections and Pyelonephritis." In K. J. Isselbacher and others (eds.), *Harrison's Principles of Internal Medicine.* (13th ed.) New York: McGraw-Hill, 1994.

Witschi, J. C., Kowaloff, H. B., and Slack, W. V. "An Interactive Dietary Interview for Hospital Employees." *M.D. Computing,* 1993, *104,* 216–224.

Witschi, J., Porter, D., Vogel, S., Buxbaum, R., Stare, F. J., and Slack, W. "A Computer-Based Dietary Counseling System." *Journal of the American Dietetic Association,* 1976, *69,* 385–390.

Chapter Four (Cybermedicine in Psychology and Psychiatry)

Bachofen, M., Nakagaw, A., Marks, I. M., Park, J. M., Greist, J. H., Baer, L., Wenzel, K. W., Parkin, J. R., and Dottl, S. L. "Home Self-Assessment and Self-Treatment of Obsessive-Compulsive Disorder Using a Manual and a Computer-Conducted Telephone Interview: Replication of a UK-US Study." *Journal of Clinical Psychiatry,* 1999, *60*(8), 545–549.

Baer, L., Brown-Beasley, M. W., Sorce, J., and Henriques, A. I. "Computer-Assisted Telephone Administration of a Structured Interview for Obsessive-Compulsive Disorder." *American Journal of Psychiatry,* 1993, *150*(11), 1737–1738.

Baer, L., and Greist, J. H. "An Interactive Computer-Administered Self-Assessment and Self-Help Program for Behavior Therapy." *Journal of Clinical Psychiatry,* 1997, *58 Supplement,* 12, 23–28.

Beck, A. T., Rush, A. J., Shaw, B. F., and Emery, G. *Cognitive Therapy of Depression.* New York: Guilford Press, 1979.

Bergeron, B., and Locke, S. E. "Speech Recognition as a User Interface." *M.D. Computing,* 1990, *6*(1), 329–334.

Berne, E. *Transactional Analysis in Psychotherapy.* New York: Grove Press, 1961.

Blood, G. W. "A Behavioral-Cognitive Therapy Program for Adults Who Stutter: Computers and Counseling." *Journal of Communication Disorders,* 1995, *28*(2), 165–185.

Bloom, S., White, R., Beckley, R., and Slack, W. "Converse: A Means to Write, Edit, Administer and Summarize Computer-Based Dialogue." *Computers and Biomedical Research,* 1978, *11,* 167–175.

Campbell, D. T., and Stanley, J. C. *Experimental and Quasi-Experimental Designs for Research.* Chicago: Rand McNally, 1963.

Carr, A. C., Ghosh, A., and Aneill, R. J. "Can a Computer Take a Psychiatric History?" *Psychological Medicine,* 1983, *13,* 151–158.

Clark, W. A., and Molnar, C. E. "A Description of the LINC." In R. W. Stacy and B. D. Waxman (eds.), *Computers in Biomedical Research.* Vol. 2. New York: Academic Press, 1965.

Coddington, R. D., and King, T. L. "Automated History Taking in Child Psychiatry." *American Journal of Psychiatry,* 1972, *129,* 52–58.

Colby, K. M., Watt, J. B., and Gilbert, J. P. "A Computer Method of Psychotherapy: Preliminary Communication." *Journal of Nervous and Mental Diseases,* 1966, *142,* 148–152.

Devine, E. G., Gaehde, S. A., and Curtis, A. C. "Comparative Evaluation of Three Continuous Speech Recognition Software Packages in the Generation of Medical Reports." *Journal of the American Medical Informatics Association,* 2000, *7,* 462–468.

Dinoff, M., Clark, C. G., Reitman, L. M., and Smith, R. E. "The Feasibility of Videotape Interviewing." *Psychological Reports,* 1969, *25,* 239–242.

Ellis, A. "The Essence of Rational Therapy." In B. N. Ard Jr. (ed.), *Counseling and Psychotherapy: Classics on Theories and Issues.* Palo Alto, Calif.: Science and Behavior Books, 1966.

Erdman, H. P., Klein, M. H., and Greist, J. H. "Direct Patient Computer Interviewing." *Journal of Consulting and Clinical Psychology,* 1985, *53,* 760–773.

Freud, S. *A General Introduction to Psychoanalysis.* (J. Riviere, trans.). New York: Pocket Books, 1921.

Fulton, S. M. "Speak Softly, Carry a Big Chip: Using Speech Recognition Software Takes Patience and Computer Power." *New York Times,* Mar. 30, 2000. Available on-line: http://www.out-loud.com.

Galanter M., Keller, D. S., Dermatis, H., and Biderman, D. "Use of the Internet for Addiction Education: Combining Network Therapy with Pharmacotherapy." *American Journal of Addiction,* 1998, *7,* 7–13.

Gendlin, E. T. *Experiencing and the Creation of Meaning.* New York: Free Press, 1962.

Glasser, W. "Reality Therapy: A Realistic Approach to the Young Offender." In B. N. Ard Jr. (ed.), *Counseling and Psychotherapy: Classics on Theories and Issues.* Palo Alto, Calif.: Science and Behavior Books, 1966.

Gould, R. L. "The Use of Computers in Therapy." In T. Trabin and M. A. Freeman (eds.), *The Computerization of Behavioral Healthcare: How to Enhance Clinical Practice, Management, and Communications.* San Francisco: Jossey-Bass, 1996.

Greist, J. H. "Computer Interviews for Depression Management." *Journal of Clinical Psychiatry,* 1998, *59 Supplement,* 16, 40–42.

Greist, J. H., Gustafson, D. H., Erdman, H. P., Taves, J. E., Klein, M. H., and Speidel, S. D. "Suicide Risk Prediction by Computer Interview: A Prospective Study." *American Journal of Psychiatry,* 1973, *130,* 1327–1332.

Greist, J. H., and Klein, M. H. "Computer Programs for Patients, Clinicians, and Researchers in Psychiatry." In J. B. Sidowski, J. H. Johnson, and T. A. Williams (eds.), *Technology in Mental Health Care Delivery Systems.* Norwood, N.J.: Ablex, 1980.

Greist, J. H., Klein, M. H., and Van Cura, L. J. "A Computer Interview for Psychiatric Patient Target Symptoms." *Archives of General Psychiatry,* 1973, *29,* 247–253.

Hofmann, M., Hock, C., and Muller-Spahn, F. "Computer-Based Cognitive Training in Alzheimer's Disease Patients." *Annals of the New York Academy of Science,* 1996, *777,* 249–254.

Jerome, L. W., DeLeon, P. H., James, L. C., Folen, R., Earles, J., and Gedney, J. J. "The Coming of Age of Telecommunications in Psychological Research and Practice." *American Psychologist,* 2000, *55,* 407–421.

Lange, A., van de Ven, J. P., Schrieken, B. A., Bredeweg, B., and Emmelkamp, P. M. "Internet-Mediated, Protocol-Driven Treatment of Psychological Dysfunction." *Journal of Telemedicine Telecare,* 2000, *6*(1), 15–21.

Lessler, J. T., and O'Reilly, J. M. "Mode of Interview and Reporting of Sensitive Issues: Design and Implementation of Audio Computer-Assisted Self-Interviewing." In *NIDA Research Monograph.* Research Triangle Institute, N.C., 1997.

Locke, S., Kowaloff, H. B., Hoff, R. G., Safran, C., Popovsky, M. A., Cotton, D. J., Finkelstein, D. M., Page, P. L., and Slack, W. V. "Computer-Based Interview for Screening Blood Donors for Risk of HIV Transmission." *Journal of the American Medical Association,* 1992, *268,* 1301–1305.

Lucas, R. W., Mullin, P. J., Luna, C.B.X., and McInroy, D. C. "Psychiatrists and a Computer as Interrogators of Patients with Alcohol-Related Illnesses: A Comparison." *British Journal of Psychiatry,* 1977, *131,* 160–167.

Marks, I. M., O'Dwyer, A. M., Meehan, O., Greist, J. H., Baer, L., and McGuire, P. "Subjective Imagery in Obsessive-Compulsive Disorder Before and After Exposure Therapy. Pilot Randomized Controlled Trial." *British Journal of Psychiatry,* 2000, *176,* 387–391.

Maultsby, M. C. *Rational Behavior Therapy.* Englewood Cliffs, N.J.: Prentice Hall, 1984.

Maultsby, M. C., and Slack, W. V. "A Computer-Based Psychiatry History System." *Archives of General Psychiatry,* 1971, *25,* 570–572.

Metzger, D. S., Koblin, B., Turner, C., Navaline, H., Valenti, F., Holte, S., Gross, M., Sheon, A., Miller, H., Cooley, P., and Seage, G. R., III. "Randomized Controlled Trial of Audio Computer-Assisted Self-

Interviewing: Utility and Acceptability in Longitudinal Studies. HIVNET Vaccine Preparedness Study Protocol Team." *American Journal of Epidemiology,* 2000, *152,* 99–106.

Millstein, S. G., and Irwin, C. E., Jr. "Acceptability of Computer-Acquired Sexual Histories in Adolescent Girls." *Journal of Pediatrics,* 1983, *103,* 815–819.

Mora, G. "History of Psychiatry." In H. I. Kaplan and B. J. Sadock (eds.), *Comprehensive Textbook of Psychiatry.* (4th ed.) Baltimore: Williams & Wilkins, 1985.

Osgood-Hynes, D. J., Greist, J. H., Marks, I. M., Baer, L., Heneman, S. W., Wenzel, K. W., Manzo, P. A., Parkin, J. R., Spierings, C. J., Dottl, S. L., and Vitse, H. M. "Self-Administered Psychotherapy for Depression Using a Telephone-Accessed Computer System Plus Booklets: An Open U.S.-U.K. Study." *Journal of Clinical Psychiatry,* 1998, *59*(7), 358–365.

Osser, D. N. "Algorithms for the Pharmacotherapy of Depression: Part One and Part Two. *Directions in Psychiatry,* 1998, *18*(3–4), 303–336.

Pearson, J. S., Rome, H. P., Swenson, W. M., Mataya, P., and Brannick, T. L. "Development of a Computer System for Scoring and Interpretation of Minnesota Multiphasic Personality Inventories in a Medical Clinic." *Annals of the New York Academy of Science,* 1965, *126*(2), 684–695.

Rogers, C. R. *Client-Centered Therapy.* Boston: Houghton Mifflin, 1965.

Rosenthal, R. *Experimenter Effects in Behavioral Research.* Englewood Cliffs, N.J.: Appleton-Century-Crofts, 1966.

Rothbaum, B. O., and Hodges, L. F. "Virtual Reality Exposure Therapy." *Journal of Psychotherapy Practice Research,* 1997, *6*(3), 219–226.

Rothbaum, B. O., and Hodges, L. F. "The Use of Virtual Reality Exposure in the Treatment of Anxiety Disorders." *Behavior Modification,* 1999, *23*(4), 507–525.

Rothbaum, B. O., Hodges, L. F., Kooper, R., Opdyke, D., Williford, J. S., and North, M. "Effectiveness of Computer-Generated (Virtual Reality) Graded Exposure in the Treatment of Acrophobia." *American Journal of Psychiatry,* 1995, *153*(4), 626–628.

Seemann, O., Seemann, M. D., Boerner, R., Jenn, M., Rupprecht, R., and Soyka, M. "Psybertherapy on the Internet and Its Implications for Psychiatry, Psychotherapy, and Psychosomatics." *European Journal of Medical Research,* 1998, *3,* 571–576.

Selmi, P. M., Klein, M. H., Greist, J. H., Sorrell, S. P., and Erdman, H. P. "Computer-Administered Cognitive-Behavioral Therapy for Depression." *American Journal of Psychiatry,* 1990, *147*(1), 51–56.

Sheridan, T. B., and Zeltzer, D. "Virtual Environments." *M.D. Computing,* 1994, *11*(5), 307–310.

Skinner, B. F. *Science and Human Behavior.* New York: Macmillan, 1953.

Skinner, H. A., and Allen, B. A. "Does the Computer Make a Difference? Computerized Versus Face-to-Face Versus Self-Report Assessment of Alcohol, Drug, and Tobacco Use." *Journal of Consulting and Clinical Psychology,* 1983, *51*(2), 267–275.

Slack, C. W. "Experimenter-Subject Psychotherapy: A New Method of Introducing Intensive Office Treatment for Unreachable Cases." *Mental Hygiene,* 1960, *44,* 238–256.

Slack, C. W. *Timothy Leary, the Madness of the Sixties and Me.* New York: Wyden, 1973.

Slack, C. W., and Slack, W. V. "Good! We Are Listening to You Talk About Your Sadness." *Psychology Today,* 1974, *7,* 62–65.

Slack, W. "Computer-Based Interviewing System Dealing with Nonverbal Behavior As Well As Keyboard Responses." *Science,* 1971, *171,* 84–87.

Slack, W. V. "Patient Counseling by Computer." In S. Zoog and S. Yarnall (eds.), *The Changing Health Care Team.* Seattle: Medical Communications and Services Association, 1976.

Slack, W. V., Leviton, A., Bennett, S. E., Fleischmann, K. H., and Lawrence, R. S. "Relation Between Age, Education, and Time to Respond to Questions in a Computer-Based Medical Interview." *Computers and Biomedical Research,* 1988, *21,* 78–84.

Slack, W. V., Porter, D., Balkin, P., Kowaloff, H. B., and Slack, C. W. "Computer-Assisted Soliloquy as an Approach to Psychotherapy." *M.D. Computing,* 1990, *7*(1), 37–58.

Slack, W. V., and Slack, C. W. "Patient-Computer Dialogue." *New England Journal of Medicine,* 1972, *286,* 1304–1309.

Slack, W. V., and Slack, C. W. "Talking to a Computer About Emotional Problems: A Comparative Study." *Psychotherapy Theory Research and Practice,* 1977, *14,* 156–164.

Spielberger, C. D., Gorsuch, R. L., and Lushene, R. E. *STAI Manual for the State-Trait Anxiety Inventory ("Self-Evaluation Questionnaire").* Palo Alto, Calif.: Consulting Psychologists Press, 1970.

Taylor, J. A. "A Personality Scale of Manifest Anxiety." *Journal of Abnormal Social Psychology,* 1953, *48,* 285–290.

Turner, C. F., Ku, L., Rogers, S. M., Lindberg, L. D., Pleck, J. H., and Sonenstein, F. L. "Adolescent Sexual Behavior, Drug Use, and Violence: Increased Reporting with Computer Survey Technology." *Science,* 1998, *280*(5365), 867–873.

Wald, J. S., Rind, D., Safran, C., Kowaloff, H., Barker, R., and Slack, W. V. "Patient Entries in the Electronic Medical Record: An Interactive Interview Used in Primary Care." In R. M. Gardner (ed.), *American Medical Informatics Association: The Proceedings of the Nineteenth Annual Symposium on Computer Applications in Medical Care.* Philadelphia: Hanley & Belfus, 1995.

Watson, J. B. *Behaviorism.* New York: Norton, 1924.

Webb, J. T. "Interview Synchrony: An Investigation of Two Speech Measures in an Automated Standardized Interview." In A. W. Siegman and R.A.B Pope (eds.), *Studies in Dyadic Communication.* New York: Pergamon Press, 1972.

Weizenbaum, J. *Computer Power and Human Reason.* New York: Freeman, 1976.

Chapter Five (The Patient On-Line)

Cyber Dialogue. "On-line Health Reaches Critical Mass." *Nua Internet Surveys 1998.* Available on-line: http://www.nua.ie/surveys.

Eng, T. R., Maxfield, A., Paatrick, K., Deering, M. J., Ratzan, S. C., and Gustafson, D. H. "Access to Health Information and Support: A Public Highway or a Private Road?" *Journal of the American Medical Association,* 1998, *280,* 1371–1375.

Ferguson, T. *Health On-line: How to Find Health Information, Support Groups, and Self-Help Communities in Cyberspace.* Reading, Mass.: Addison-Wesley, 1996.

Ferguson, T. "Digital Doctoring: Opportunities and Challenges in Electronic Patient-Physician Communication." *Journal of the American Medical Association,* 1998, *280,* 1361–1362.

Ferguson, T. "Online Patient-Helpers and Physicians Working Together: A New Partnership for High Quality Health Care." *British Medical Journal,* 2000, *321,* 1129–1132.

Ferguson, T. *The Ferguson Report.* Available on-line: http://www.ferguson-report.com.

Fox, S., and Rainie, L. "The Online Health Care Revolution: How the Web Helps Americans Take Better Care of Themselves." *Pew Internet & American Life Project, 2000.* Available on-line: http://www.pewinternet.org.

Frisse, M. E., Kelly, E. A., and Metcalfe, E. S. "An Internet Primer: Resources and Responsibilities." *Academic Medicine,* 1994, *69,* 20–24.

Gralla, P. *How the Internet Works.* Indianapolis: QUE, 1999.

Hahn, H., and Stout, R. *The Internet Complete Reference.* New York: McGraw-Hill, 1994.

Kehoe, B. P. *Zen and the Art of the Internet: A Beginner's Guide.* (3rd ed.) Englewood Cliffs, N.J.: Prentice Hall, 1994.

Krol, E. *The Whole Internet User's Guide and Catalog.* (2nd ed.) Sebastopol, Calif.: O'Reilly, 1994.

Levine, J. R., and Baroudi, C. *The Internet for Dummies.* San Mateo, Calif.: IDG Books Worldwide, 1993.

Louis Harris & Associates. "Sixty Million Seek Health Info On-line in the US." *Nua Internet Surveys 1999.* Available on-line: http://www.nua.ie/surveys.

"Medical Hardware and Software Buyers Guide." *M.D. Computing,* 1996, *13*(6), 486–576.

Nua. "How Many On-line?" *Nua Internet Surveys 2000.* Available on-line: http://www.nua.ie/surveys.

O'Neil, J. "Health Care Online and in the Third Person." *New York Times,* Dec. 19, 2000. Available on-line: http://www.nytimes.com.

Orzack, M. H. "How to Recognize and Treat Computer.com Addictions." *Directions in Clinical and Counseling Psychology. Lesson 2.* New York: Hatherleigh, 1999.

Pannen, M. "Guide to the Internet: The World Wide Web." *British Medical Journal,* 1995, *311*, 1552–1556.

Rogers, C. R. *Client-Centered Therapy.* Boston: Houghton Mifflin, 1965.

Scolamiero, S. J. "Support Groups in Cyberspace." *M.D. Computing,* 1996, *14*(1), 12–17.

Slack C. W., Porter D., Slack W. V. "Some Nostalgic Reflections on Computer-Assisted Instruction." In E. C. Deland (ed.), *Computers in Biomedical Education.* New York: Plenum, 1978.

Slack, W. V. "The Handheld Calculator." *M.D. Computing,* 1991, *8*(1), 8–10.

Zelingher, J. "Exploring the Internet." *M.D. Computing,* 1995, *12*(2), 100–108.

Chapter Six (Cybermedicine in the Hospital and Clinic)

Aller, R. D., Robboy, S. J., Poitras, J. W., Altshuler, B. S., Cameron, M., Prior, M. C., Miao, S., and Barnett, G. O. "Computer-Assisted Pathology Encoding and Reporting System (CAPER)." *American Journal of Clinical Pathology,* 1977, *68*, 715–720.

Anderson, J. G., and Jay, S. J. *Use and Impact of Computers in Clinical Medicine.* New York: Springer-Verlag, 1987.

Bakker, A. R. "The Development of an Integrated and Co-Operative Hospital Information System." *Medical Informatics (London)*, 1984, *9*, 135–142.

Ball, M. J., Douglas, J. V., O'Desky, R. I., and Albright, J. W. *Healthcare Information Management Systems: A Practical Guide*. New York: Springer-Verlag, 1991.

Barnett, G. O. "The Application of Computer-Based Medical Record Systems in Ambulatory Practice." *New England Journal of Medicine*, 1984, *9*, 135–142.

Bleich, H. L. "The Kaiser Permanente Health Plan, Dr. Morris F. Collen, and Automated Multiphasic Testing." *M.D. Computing*, 1994, *11*(3), 136–139.

Bleich, H. L., Beckley, R. F., Horowitz, G., Jackson, J., Moody, E., Franklin, C., Goodman, S. R., McKay, M. W., Pope, R. A., Walden, T., Bloom, S. A., and Slack, W. V. "Clinical Computing in a Teaching Hospital." *New England Journal of Medicine*, 1985, *312*(12), 756–764.

Bleich, H. L., Safran, C., and Slack, W. V. "Departmental and Laboratory Computing in Two Hospitals." *M.D. Computing*, 1989, *6*(3), 149–155.

Bleich, H. L., and Slack, W. V. "Clinical Computing." *M.D. Computing*, 1989, *6*(3), 132–135.

Bleich, H. L., and Slack, W. V. "Designing a Hospital Information System: A Comparison of Interfaced and Integrated Systems." *M.D. Computing*, 1992, *9*(5), 293–296.

Boro, E. S. "Different Drummers: Neil Pappalardo." *M.D. Computing*, 1990, *7*, 326–327.

Clayton, P. D., Sideli, R. V., and Sengupta, S. "Open Architecture and Integrated Information at Columbia-Presbyterian Medical Center." *M.D. Computing*, 1992, *9*(5), 297–303.

Colby, K. M., Watt, J. B., and Gilbert, J. P. "A Computer Method of Psychotherapy: Preliminary Communication." *Journal of Nervous and Mental Diseases*, 1966, *142*, 148–152.

Collen, M. F. "The Multitest Laboratory in Health Care of the Future." *Hospitals*, 1967, *41*, 119–125.

Collen, M. F. *A History of Medical Informatics in the United States, 1950 to 1990*. Bethesda, Md.: American Medical Informatics Association, 1995.

Collen, M. F., Rubin, L., Neyman, J., Dantzig, G. B., Baer R. M., and Siegelaub, A. B. "Automated Multiphasic Screening and Diagnosis." *American Journal of Public Health*, 1964, *54*, 741–750.

Devine, E. G., Gaehde, S. A., and Curtis, A. C. "Comparative Evaluation of Three Continuous Speech Recognition Software Packages in the Generation of Medical Reports." *Journal of the American Medical Informatics Association,* 2000, *7,* 462–468.

Feinstein, A. R. *Clinical Judgment.* Baltimore, Md.: Williams & Wilkins, 1967.

Freudenheim, M. "Digital Doctoring." *New York Times,* Jan. 8, 2001 (www.nytimes.com).

Gardner, R. M. "Collaboration in Clinical Computing at LDS Hospital." *M.D. Computing,* 1994, *11*(1), 10–13.

Glaser, J. P., Beckley, R. F., III, Roberts, P., Mara, J. K., Hiltz, F. L., and Hurley, J. "A Very Large PC LAN as the Basis for a Hospital Information System." *Journal of Medical Systems,* 1991, *15*(2), 133–137.

Gouveia, W. A., Diamantis, C., and Barnett, G. O. "Computer Applications in the Hospital Medication System." *American Journal of Hospital Pharmacy,* 1969, *26,* 140–150.

Greenes, R. A., Pappalardo, A. N., Marble, C. W., and Barnett, G. O. "Design and Implementation of a Clinical Data Management System." *Computers and Biomedical Research,* 1969, *2,* 469–485.

Greenes, R. A., and Shortliffe, E. H. "Medical Informatics: An Emerging Academic Discipline and Institutional Priority." *Journal of the American Medical Association,* 1990, *263,* 1114–1120.

Grossman, J. H., Barnett, G. O., Koepsell, T. D., Nesson H. R., Dorsey, J. L., and Phillips, R. R. "An Automated Medical Record System." *Journal of the American Medical Association,* 1973, *224,* 1616–1621.

Hadley, T. P., Geer, D. E., Bleich, H. L., and Freedberg, I. M. "The Use of Digital Computers in Dermatological Diagnosis: Computer-Aided Diagnosis of Febrile Illness with Eruption." *Journal of Investigative Dermatology,* 1974, *62,* 467–472.

Halacy, D. S. *Computers: The Machines We Think With.* New York: Dell, 1962.

Hammond, W. E. "The Status of Healthcare Standards in the United States." *International Journal of Biomedical Computing,* 1995, *39,* 87–92.

Hendrickson, G., Anderson, R. K., Clayton, P. D., Cimino, J., Hripcsak, G. M., Johnson, S. B., McCormack, M., Sengupta, S., Shea, S., Sideli, R., and Roderer, N. "The Integrated Academic Information Management System at Columbia-Presbyterian Medical Center." *M.D. Computing,* 1992, *9*(1), 35–42.

Hicks, G. P., Gieschen, M. M., Slack, W. V., and Larson, F. C. "Routine Use of a Small Digital Computer in the Clinical Laboratory." *Journal of the American Medical Association,* 1966, *196,* 973–978.

Jacquez, J. A. (ed.). *The Diagnostic Process: Proceedings of Conference Held at the University of Michigan.* Ann Arbor, Mich.: Malloy Lithographing, 1964.

Jacquez, J. A. (ed.). *Computer Diagnosis and Diagnostic Methods: The Proceedings of the Second Conference on the Diagnostic Process Held at the University of Michigan.* Springfield, Ill.: Thomas, 1972.

Karpinski, R. H., and Bleich, H. L. "MISAR: A Miniature Information Storage and Retrieval System." *Computers and Biomedical Research,* 1971, *4,* 655–660.

Kim, I. "Handheld Calculators: Functions at the Fingertips." *Mechanical Engineering,* 1990, *112,* 56–62.

Ledley, R. S., and Lusted, L. B. "Reasoning Foundations of Medical Diagnosis." *Science,* 1959, *130,* 9–21.

Leeming, B. W., Simon, M., Jackson, J. D., Horowitz, G. L., and Bleich, H. L. "Advances in Radiological Reporting Computerized Language Information Processing (CLIP)." *Radiology,* 1979, *133*(2), 349–353.

Lindberg, D. A. "Collection, Evaluation, and Transmission of Hospital Laboratory Data." *Methods of Information in Medicine,* 1967, *6,* 97–107.

Lindberg, D. A., and Humphreys, B. L. "Computers in Medicine." *Journal of the American Medical Association,* 1995, *273,* 1667–1668.

Lipkin, M., Engle, R. L., Jr., Flehinger, B. J., Gerstman, L. J., and Atamer, M. A. "Computer-Aided Differential Diagnosis of Hematological Diseases." *Annals of the New York Academy of Science,* 1969, *161,* 670–679.

Lodwick, G. S., Turner, A. H., Lusted, L. B., and Templeton, A. W. "Computer-Aided Analysis of Radiographic Images." *Journal of Chronic Disease,* 1966, *19,* 485–496.

Lusted, L. B. *Introduction to Medical Decision Making.* Springfield, Ill.: Thomas, 1968.

McDonald, C. J., Murray, R., Jeris, D., Bhargave, B., Seeger, J., and Blevins, L. "A Computer-Based Record and Clinical Monitoring System for Ambulatory Care." *American Journal of Public Health,* 1977, *67,* 240–245.

McDonald, C. J., Tierney, W. M., Overhage, J. M., Martin, D. K., and Wilson, G. "The Regenstrief Medical Record System: 20 Years of Experience in Hospitals, Clinics, and Neighborhood Health Centers." *M.D. Computing,* 1992, *9*(4), 206–218.

Melski, J. W., Geer, D. E., and Bleich, H. L. "Medical Information Storage and Retrieval Using Preprocessed Variables." *Computers and Biomedical Research,* 1978, *11,* 613–621.

Orthner, H. F., and Blum, B. I. *Implementing Health Care Information Systems.* New York: Springer-Verlag, 1989.

Pauker, S. G., and Kassirer, J. P. "Therapeutic Decision Making: A Cost-Benefit Analysis." *New England Journal of Medicine,* 1975, *293,* 229–234.

Pope, R. A., Mattson, C. J., Janousek, J., and Slack, W. V. "A Computer-Based IV Admixture System." *Methods of Information in Medicine,* 1982, *21*(2), 65–69.

Pryor, T. A., Gardner, R. M., Clayton, P. D., and Warner, H. R. "The HELP System." *Journal of Medical Systems,* 1983, *7,* 87–102.

Reich, P. R., Geer, D. E., and Bleich, H. L. "A Computer Program for the Diagnosis of Hematological Disorders." *American Journal of Hematology,* 1977, *3,* 127–135.

Safran, C., Porter, D., Slack, W. V., and Bleich, H. L. "Diagnosis-Related Groups: A Critical Assessment of the Provision for Comorbidity." *Medical Care,* 1987, *25,* 1011–1014.

Safran, C., Slack, W. V., and Bleich, H. L. "Role of Computing in Patient Care in Two Hospitals." *M.D. Computing,* 1989, *6*(3), 141–148.

Scherrer, J. R., Baud, R. H., Hochstrasser, D., and Ratib, O. "An Integrated Hospital Information System in Geneva." *M.D. Computing,* 1990, *7*(2), 81–89.

Schwartz, W. B. "Medicine and the Computer: The Promise and Problems of Change." *New England Journal of Medicine,* 1970, *283,* 1257–1264.

Schwartz, W. B., Patil, R. S., and Szolovits, P. "Artificial Intelligence in Medicine: Where Do We Stand?" *New England Journal of Medicine,* 1987, *316,* 685–688.

Shelley, M. W. *Frankenstein, or, The Modern Prometheus.* New York: New American Library, 2000. (Originally published 1818.)

Shortliffe, E. H., Davis, R., Axline, S. G., Buchanan, B. G., Green, C. C., and Cohen, S. N. "Computer-Based Consultations in Clinical Therapeutics: Explanation and Rule Acquisition Capabilities of the MYCIN System." *Computers and Biomedical Research,* 1975, *8,* 303–320.

Shortliffe, E. H., and Perreault, L. E. (eds.) with Wiederhold, G., and Fagan, L. M. (assoc. eds.). *Medical Informatics: Computer Applications in Health Care and Biomedicine.* New York: Springer-Verlag, 2000.

Simborg, D. W., Chadwick, M., Whiting O'Keefe, Q. E., Tolchin, S. G.,

Kahn, S. A., and Bergan, E. S. "Local Area Networks and the Hospital." *Computers and Biomedical Research,* 1983, *16,* 247–259.

Slack, W. V. "The Computer and the Doctor-Patient Relationship." *M.D. Computing,* 1989, *6*(6), 320–321.

Slack, W. V. "How to Become a Genius." *M.D. Computing,* 1989, *6*(5), 262–263.

Slack, W. V. "The Handheld Calculator." *M.D. Computing,* 1991, *8,* 8–10.

Slack, W. V., and Bleich, H. L. "The CCC System in Two Teaching Hospitals: A Progress Report." *International Journal of Medical Informatics,* 1999, *54,* 183–196.

Slack, W. V., Safran, C., and Bleich, H. L. "Computerization in Hospital-Based Delivery Systems." In T. Trabin and M. A. Freeman (eds.), *The Computerization of Behavioral Healthcare: How to Enhance Clinical Practice, Management, and Communications.* San Francisco: Jossey-Bass, 1996.

Slack, W. V., and Slack, C. W. "Patient-Computer Dialogue." *New England Journal of Medicine,* 1972, *286,* 1304–1309.

Stead, W. W., Borden, R., Bourne, J., Giuse, D., Biuse, N., Harris, T. R., Miller, R. A., and Olsen, A. J. "The Vanderbilt University Fast Track to IAIMS: Transition from Planning to Implementation." *Journal of the American Medical Informatics Association,* 1996, *3,* 308–317.

Stead, W. W., and Hammond, W. E. "Computerized Medical Records: A New Resource for Clinical Decision Making." *Journal of Medical Systems,* 1983, *7,* 213–220.

Szolovits, P., Patil, R. S., and Schwartz, W. B. "Artificial Intelligence in Medical Diagnosis." *Annals of Internal Medicine,* 1988, *108,* 80–87.

Warner, H. R., Olmsted, C. M., and Rutherford, B. D. "HELP: A Program for Medical Decision-Making." *Computers and Biomedical Research,* 1972, *5,* 65–74.

Warner, H. R., Toronto, A. F., Veasey, L. G., and Stephenson, R. "A Mathematical Approach to Medical Diagnosis: Application to Congenital Heart Disease." *Journal of the American Medical Association,* 1961, *177*(3), 177–183.

Weed, L. L. "Medical Records That Guide and Teach." *New England Journal of Medicine,* 1968, *278,* 593–600, 652–657.

Weed, L. L. "Technology Is a Link, Not a Barrier, for Doctor and Patient." *Modern Hospital,* 1970, *114*(2), 80–83.

Weizenbaum, J. *Computer Power and Human Reason.* New York: Freeman, 1976.

Whiting-O'Keefe, Q. E., Whiting, A., and Henke, J. "The STOR Clinical Information System." *M.D. Computing,* 1988, *5*(5), 8–21.

Chapter Seven (Cybermedicine in the Care of the Patient)

Barlam, T. F., Kowaloff, H. B., Zaleznik, D. F., Sands, K. E., and Slack, W. V. "Use of an Interactive Computer Program for Universal Precaution Training." Manuscript in preparation.

Bates, D. W., Kuperman, G. J., Rittenberg, E., Teich, J. M., Fiskio, J., Ma'luf, N., Onderdonk, A., Wybenga, D., Winkelman, J., Brennan, T. A., Komaroff, A. L., and Tanasijevic, M. "A Randomized Trial of a Computer-Based Intervention to Reduce Utilization of Redundant Laboratory Tests." *American Journal of Medicine,* 1999, *106*, 144–150.

Bates, D. W., Teich, J. M., Lee, J., Seger, D., Kuperman, G. J., Ma'Luf, N., Boyle, D., and Leape, L. "The Impact of Computerized Physician Order Entry on Medication Error Prevention." *Journal of the American Medical Informatics Association,* 1999, *6*, 313–321.

Bleich, H. L. "The Computer as a Consultant." *New England Journal of Medicine,* 1971, *284*, 141–147.

Bleich, H. L., Beckley, R. F., Horowitz, G., Jackson, J., Moody, E., Franklin, C., Goodman, S. R., McKay, M. W., Pope, R. A., Walden, T., Bloom, S. A., and Slack, W. V. "Clinical Computing in a Teaching Hospital." *New England Journal of Medicine,* 1985, *312*(12), 756–764.

Bleich, H. L., Safran, C., and Slack, W. V. "Departmental and Laboratory Computing in Two Hospitals." *M.D. Computing,* 1989, *6*(3), 149–155.

Bloom, S., White, R., Beckley, R., and Slack, W. "Converse: A Means to Write, Edit, Administer and Summarize Computer-Based Dialogue." *Computers and Biomedical Research,* 1978, *11*, 167–175.

Bourie, P. Q., Chapman, R. H., Dai, S., and Reiley, P. "An Automated Nursing Assessment for a Teaching Hospital." *M.D. Computing,* 1997, *14*(1), 57–60.

Degoulet, P., Chatellier, G., Devries, V., Lavril, M., and Menard, J. "Computer-Assisted Techniques for Evaluation of Hypertensive Patients." *American Journal of Hypertension,* 1990, *3*, 156–163.

Devine, E. G., Gaehde, S. A., and Curtis, A. C. "Comparative Evaluation of Three Continuous Speech Recognition Software Packages in the Generation of Medical Reports." *Journal of the American Medical Informatics Association,* 2000, *7*, 462–468.

Einbinder, J. S., Rury, C., and Safran, C. "Outcomes Research Using the

Electronic Patient Record: Beth Israel Hospital's Experience with Anticoagulation." In R. M. Gardner (ed.), *American Medical Informatics Association: The Proceedings of the Nineteenth Annual Symposium on Computer Applications in Medical Care.* Philadelphia: Hanley & Belfus, 1995.

Fordham, D., McPhee, S. J., Bird, J. A., Rodnick, J. E., and Detmer, W. M. "The Cancer Prevention Reminder System." *M.D. Computing,* 1990, *7*(5), 289–295.

Frame, P. S. "Can Computerized Reminder Systems Have an Impact on Preventive Services in Practice?" *Journal of General Internal Medicine,* 1990, *Supplement 5,* S112-S115.

Herrmann, F. R., Safran, C., Levkoff, S. E., and Minaker, K. L. "Serum Albumin Level on Admission as a Predictor of Death, Length of Stay, and Readmission." *Archives of Internal Medicine,* 1992, *152,* 125–130.

Horowitz, G. L., and Bleich, H. L. "PaperChase: A Computer Program to Search the Medical Literature." *New England Journal of Medicine,* 1981, *305,* 924–930.

Kuperman, G. J., Boyle, D., Jha, A., Rittenberg, E., Ma'Luf, N., Tanasijevic, M. J., Teich, J. M., Winkelman, J., and Bates, D. W. "How Promptly Are Inpatients Treated for Critical Laboratory Results?" *Journal of the American Medical Informatics Association,* 1998, *5,* 112–119.

Kuperman, G. J., Teich, J. M., Bates, D. W., Hiltz, F. L., Hurley, J. M., Lee, R. Y., and Paterno, M. D. "Detecting Alerts, Notifying the Physician, and Offering Action Items: A Comprehensive Alerting System." In J. J. Cimino (ed.), *A Symposium of the American Medical Informatics Association, October 26–30, 1996.* Philadelphia: Hanley & Belfus, 1996.

Landro, L. ". . . Deal with Our Doctors: Two Boston Hospital Groups Are Showing How Technology Can Heal More Than the Bottom Line." *Wall Street Journal,* Nov. 13, 2000, p. R23.

McCarty, R. J., Kanter, T., and Sopanen, J. *Lifeline.* Videotape documentary of clinical computing systems developed for Boston's Beth Israel and Brigham and Women's hospitals by the Center for Clinical Computing. Produced by RJM Associates, 1995.

McCarty, R. J., Kanter, T., and Sopanen, J. Video archives of interviews of users and developers of cybermedicine systems in Beth Israel and Brigham and Women's hospitals. Produced by RJM Associates, 1995.

McDonald, C. J. "Protocol-Based Computer Reminders, the Quality of Care and the Non-Perfectibility of Man." *New England Journal of Medicine,* 1976, *295*(24), 1351–1355.

McDonald, C. J., Wilson, G. A., and McCabe, G. P. "Physician Response to Computer Reminders." *Journal of the American Medical Association,* 1980, *244,* 1579–1581.

Mok, M. P., Castile, J. A., Kowaloff, H. B., and Janousek, J. R. "Drugman: A Computerized Supplement to a Hospital's Drug Information Newsletter." *American Journal of Hospital Pharmacy,* 1985, *42,* 1565–1567.

Ornstein, S. M., Garr, D. R., Jenkins, R. G., Rust, P. F., and Arnon, A. "Computer-Generated Physician and Patient Reminders: Tools to Improve Population Adherence to Selected Preventive Services." *Journal of Family Practice,* 1991, *32,* 82–90.

Pauker, S. G., Gorry, G. A., Kassirer, J. P., and Schwartz, W. B. "Towards the Simulation of Clinical Cognition: Taking a Present Illness by Computer." *American Journal of Medicine,* 1976, *60,* 981–996.

Pauker, S. G., and Kassirer, J. P. "Therapeutic Decision Making: A Cost-Benefit Analysis." *New England Journal of Medicine,* 1975, *293,* 229–234.

Physicians' Desk Reference. Montvale, N.J.: Medical Economics, 1996.

Rind, D. M., Safran, C., Phillips, R. S., Wang, Q., Calkins, D. R., Delbanco, T. L., Bleich, H. L., and Slack, W. V. "Effect of Computer-Based Alerts on the Treatment and Outcomes of Hospitalized Patients." *Archives of Internal Medicine,* 1994, *154,* 1511–1517.

Safran, C., Herrmann, F., Rind, D., Kowaloff, H., Bleich, H., and Slack, W. V. "Computer-Based Support for Clinical Decision Making." *M.D. Computing,* 1990, *7*(5), 319–322.

Safran, C., Porter, D., Lightfoot, J., Rury, C. D., Underhill, L. H., Bleich, H. L., and Slack, W. V. "ClinQuery: A System for On-line Searching of Data in a Teaching Hospital." *Annals of Internal Medicine,* 1989, *9,* 751–756.

Safran, C., Rind, D. M., Davis, R. B., Ives, D., Sands, D. Z., Currier, J., Slack, W. V., Makadon, H. J., and Cotton, D. J. "Guidelines for Management of HIV Infection with Computer-Based Patient's Record." *Lancet,* 1995, *346,* 341–346.

Safran, C., Rury, C., Rind, D. M., and Taylor, W. C. "A Computer-Based Ambulatory Medical Record for a Teaching Hospital." *M.D. Computing,* 1991, *8*(5), 291–299.

Safran, C., Slack, W. V., and Bleich, H. L. "Role of Computing in Patient Care in Two Hospitals." *M.D. Computing,* 1989, *6*(3), 141–148.

Sands, D. Z., and Safran, C. "Enhancing Patient Care with Computerized Clinical Formulas." *Clinical Research,* 1993, *41,* 527A.

Sands, D. Z., Safran, C., Slack, W. V., and Bleich, H. L. "Use of E-Mail in a Teaching Hospital." In *Seventeenth Annual Symposium on Computer Applications in Medical Care.* New York: McGraw-Hill, 1994.

Slack, W. V. "Patient Power." In J. A. Jacquez (ed.), *Computer Diagnosis and Diagnostic Methods: The Proceedings of the Second Conference on the Diagnostic Process Held at the University of Michigan.* Springfield, Ill.: Thomas, 1972.

Slack, W. V. "The Patient's Right to Decide." *Lancet,* 1977, *2,* 240.

Slack, W. V., and Bleich, H. L. "The CCC System in Two Teaching Hospitals: A Progress Report." *International Journal of Medical Informatics,* 1999, *54,* 183–196.

Slack, W. V., Peckham, B. M., Van Cura, L. J., and Carr, W. F. "A Computer-Based Physical Examination System." *Journal of the American Medical Association,* 1967, *200,* 224–228.

Slack, W. V., Safran, C., and Bleich, H. L. "Computerization in Hospital-Based Delivery Systems." In T. Trabin and M. A. Freeman (eds.), *The Computerization of Behavioral Healthcare: How to Enhance Clinical Practice, Management, and Communications.* San Francisco: Jossey-Bass, 1996.

Teich, J. M., Glaser, J. P., Beckley, R. F., Aranow, M., Bates, D. W., Kuperman, G. J., Ward, M. E., and Spurr, C. D. "The Brigham Integrated Computing System (BICS): Advanced Clinical Systems in an Academic Hospital Environment." *International Journal of Medical Informatics,* 1999, *54,* 197–208.

Tierney, W. M., McDonald, C. J., Martin, D. K., Hui, S. L., and Rogers, M. P. "Computerized Display of Past Test Results: Effect on Ambulatory Testing." *Annals of Internal Medicine,* 1987, *107,* 569–574.

Warner, H. R., Olmsted, C. M., and Rutherford, B. D. "HELP: A Program for Medical Decision-Making." *Computers and Biomedical Research,* 1972, *5,* 65–74.

Weed, L. L. "Medical Records That Guide and Teach." *New England Journal of Medicine,* 1968, *278,* 593–600, 652–657.

Weed, L. L. *Knowledge Coupling: New Premises and New Tools for Medical Care and Education.* New York: Springer-Verlag, 1991.

Weingarten, J. "Can Confidential Information Be Kept Private in High-Tech Medicine?" *M.D. Computing,* 1992, *9*(2), 79–82.

Wilson, G. A., McDonald, C. J., and McCabe, G. P., Jr. "The Effect of Immediate Access to a Computerized Medical Record on Physician Test Ordering: A Controlled Clinical Trial in the Emergency Room." *American Journal of Public Health,* 1982, *72,* 698–702.

Chapter Eight (How Well Does It Work?)

Bates, D. W., Kuperman, G. J., Rittenberg, E., Teich, J. M., Fiskio, J., Ma'luf, N., Onderdonk, A., Wybenga, D., Winkelman, J., Brennan, T. A., Komaroff, A. L., and Tanasijevic, M. "A Randomized Trial of a Computer-Based Intervention to Reduce Utilization of Redundant Laboratory Tests." *American Journal of Medicine,* 1999, *106,* 144–150.

Bates, D. W., Pappius, E., Kuperman, G. J., Sittig, D., Burstin, H., Fairchild, D., Brennan, T. A., and Teich, J. M. "Using Information Systems to Measure and Improve Quality." *International Journal of Medical Informatics,* 1999, *53,* 115–124.

Bates, D. W., Teich, J. M., Lee, J., Seger, D., Kuperman, G. J., Ma'Luf, N., Boyle, D., and Leape, L. "The Impact of Computerized Physician Order Entry on Medication Error Prevention." *Journal of the American Medical Informatics Association,* 1999, *6,* 313–321.

Berwick, D. M. "Continuous Improvement as an Ideal in Health Care." *New England Journal of Medicine,* 1989, *320,* 53–56.

Bleich, H. L. "Medical Practice and Statistical Analysis." *M.D. Computing,* 1992, *9,* 281.

Bleich, H. L., Beckley, R. F., Horowitz, G., Jackson, J., Moody, E., Franklin, C., Goodman, S. R., McKay, M. W., Pope, R. A., Walden, T., Bloom, S. A., and Slack, W. V. "Clinical Computing in a Teaching Hospital." *New England Journal of Medicine,* 1985, *312*(12), 756–764.

Bleich, H. L., Safran, C., and Slack, W. V. "Departmental and Laboratory Computing in Two Hospitals." *M.D. Computing,* 1989, *6*(3), 149–155.

Bloom, S., White, R., Beckley, R., and Slack, W. "Converse: A Means to Write, Edit, Administer and Summarize Computer-Based Dialogue." *Computers and Biomedical Research,* 1978, *11,* 167–175.

Dewey, J. *Intelligence in the Modern World.* New York: Random House, 1939.

Feinstein, A. R. *Clinical Biostatistics.* Saint Louis, Mo.: Mosby, 1977.

Hendrickson, G., Anderson, R. K., Clayton, P. D., Cimino, J., Hripcsak, G. M., Johnson, S. B., McCormack, M., Sengupta, S., Shea, S., Sideli, R., and Roderer, N. "The Integrated Academic Information Management System at Columbia-Presbyterian Medical Center." *M.D. Computing,* 1992, *9*(1), 35–42.

Horowitz, G. L., and Bleich, H. L. "PaperChase: A Computer Program to Search the Medical Literature." *New England Journal of Medicine,* 1981, *305,* 924–930.

Horowitz, G. L., Jackson, J. D., and Bleich, H. L. "PaperChase: Self-Service

Bibliographic Retrieval." *Journal of the American Medical Association,* 1983, *250*(18), 2494–2499.

Kohn, L. T., Corrigan, J. M., and Donaldson, M. S. (eds.). *To Err Is Human: Building a Safer Health System.* Institute of Medicine Committee on Quality of Health Care in America. Washington, D.C.: National Academy Press, 2000.

Kuperman, G. J., Boyle, D., Jha, A., Rittenberg, E., Ma'Luf, N., Tanasijevic, M. J., Teich, J. M., Winkelman, J., and Bates, D. W. "How Promptly Are Inpatients Treated for Critical Laboratory Results?" *Journal of the American Medical Informatics Association,* 1998, *5,* 112–119.

Kuperman, G. J., Teich, J. M., Bates, D. W., Hiltz, F. L., Hurley, J. M., Lee, R. Y., and Paterno, M. D. "Detecting Alerts, Notifying the Physician, and Offering Action Items: A Comprehensive Alerting System." In J. J. Cimino (ed.), *A Symposium of the American Medical Informatics Association,* October 26–30, 1996. Philadelphia: Hanley & Belfus, 1996.

Leape, L. L. "Institute of Medicine Medical Error Figures Are Not Exaggerated." *Journal of the American Medical Association,* 2000, *284,* 95–97.

Lindberg, D. A. "The National Library of Medicine and Its Role." *Bulletin of the Medical Library Association,* 1993, *81,* 71–73.

McDonald, C. J., Weiner, M., and Hui, S. L. "Deaths Due to Medical Errors Are Exaggerated in Institute of Medicine Report." *Journal of the American Medical Association,* 2000, *284,* 93–95.

McDonald, C. J., Wilson, G. A., and McCabe, G. P. "Physician Response to Computer Reminders." *Journal of the American Medical Association,* 1980, *244,* 1579–1581.

McKinney, W. P., Wagner, J. M., Bunton, M. S., and Kirk, L. M. "A Guide to Mosaic and the World Wide Web for Physicians." *M.D. Computing,* 1995, *12*(2), 109–114, 141.

Nicoll, N. H. "Grateful Med: An Easy to Use Information Tool." *Reflections,* 1992, *18*(3), 40–41.

Rind, D. M., Safran, C., Phillips, R. S., Wang, Q., Calkins, D. R., Delbanco, T. L., Bleich, H. L., and Slack, W. V. "Effect of Computer-Based Alerts on the Treatment and Outcomes of Hospitalized Patients." *Archives of Internal Medicine,* 1994, *154,* 1511–1517.

Rockefeller, R. G. "Onboard Medical Guidance." Health Commons Institute, 2000 (www.healthcommons.org).

Safran, C., Herrmann, F., Rind, D., Kowaloff, H. B., Bleich, H. L., and Slack, W. V. "Computer-Based Support for Clinical Decision Making." *M.D. Computing,* 1990, *7*(5), 319–322.

Safran, C., Rind, D. M., Davis, R. B., Ives, D., Sands, D. Z., Currier, J., Slack, W. V., Makadon, H. J., and Cotton, D. J. "Guidelines for Management of HIV Infection with Computer-Based Patient's Record." *Lancet,* 1995, *346,* 341–346.

Safran, C., Slack, W. V., and Bleich, H. L. "Role of Computing in Patient Care in Two Hospitals." *M.D. Computing,* 1989, *6*(3), 141–148.

Sands, D. Z., Safran, C., Slack, W. V., and Bleich, H. L. "Use of E-Mail in a Teaching Hospital." In *Seventeenth Annual Symposium on Computer Applications in Medical Care.* New York: McGraw-Hill, 1994.

Skinner, B. F. *Science and Human Behavior.* New York: Macmillan, 1953.

Slack, W. V. "Democracy and the Computer in America." *M.D. Computing,* 1992, *9*(6), 341–342.

Slack, W. V. "Assessing the Clinician's Use of Computers." *M.D. Computing,* 1993, *10*(6), 357–360.

Slack, W. V., Safran, C., and Bleich, H. L. "Computerization in Hospital-Based Delivery Systems." In T. Trabin and M. A. Freeman (eds.), *The Computerization of Behavioral Healthcare: How to Enhance Clinical Practice, Management, and Communications.* San Francisco: Jossey-Bass, 1996.

Slack, W. V., and Van Cura, L. J. "Patient Reaction to Computer-Based Medical Interviewing." *Computers and Biomedical Research,* 1968, *1,* 527–531.

Slack, W. V., Van Cura, L. J., and Greist, J. H. "Computers and Doctors: Use and Consequences." *Computers and Biomedical Research,* 1970, *3,* 521–527.

Warner, H. R., Olmsted, C. M., and Rutherford, B. D. "HELP: A Program for Medical Decision-Making." *Computers and Biomedical Research,* 1972, *5,* 65–74.

Watson, J. B. *Behaviorism.* New York: Norton, 1924.

Chapter Nine (The Clinician On-Line)

Bleich, H. L., Beckley, R. F., Horowitz, G., Jackson, J., Moody, E., Franklin, C., Goodman, S. R., McKay, M. W., Pope, R. A., Walden, T., Bloom, S. A., and Slack, W. V. "Clinical Computing in a Teaching Hospital." *New England Journal of Medicine,* 1985, *312*(12), 756–764.

Glowniak, J. V., and Bushway, M. K. "Computer Networks as a Medical Resource: Accessing and Using the Internet." *Journal of the American Medical Association,* 1994, *271,* 1934–1939.

Golden, P. A., Beauclair, R., and Sussman, L. "Factors Affecting E-Mail Use." *Computers in Human Behavior,* 1992, *8,* 297–311.

Hogarth, M. *An Internet Guide for the Health Professional.* Personal publication, mahogarth@ucdavis.edu, 1994.

Horowitz, G. L., and Bleich, H. L. "PaperChase: A Computer Program to Search the Medical Literature." *New England Journal of Medicine,* 1981, *305,* 924–930.

Horowitz, G. L., Jackson, J. D., and Bleich, H. L. "PaperChase: Self-Service Bibliographic Retrieval." *Journal of the American Medical Association,* 1983, *250*(18), 2494–2499.

McConnell, J. "Medicine on the Superhighway." *Lancet,* 1993, *342,* 1313–1314.

Nua. "Cyber Dialogue: Doctors Keep Work Offline." *Nua Internet Surveys, 2001.* Available on-line: http://www.nua.ie/surveys.

Pannen, M. "Guide to the Internet: The World Wide Web." *British Medical Journal,* 1995, *311,* 1552–1556.

Safran, C., Slack, W. V., and Bleich, H. L. "Role of Computing in Patient Care in Two Hospitals." *M.D. Computing,* 1989, *6*(3), 141–148.

Sands, D. Z., Safran, C., Slack, W. V., and Bleich, H. L. "Use of E-Mail in a Teaching Hospital." In *Seventeenth Annual Symposium on Computer Applications in Medical Care.* New York: McGraw-Hill, 1994.

Slack, W. V. "Assessing the Clinician's Use of Computers." *M.D. Computing,* 1993, *10*(6), 357–360.

Slack, W. V., Safran, C., and Bleich, H. L. "Computerization in Hospital-Based Delivery Systems." In T. Trabin and M. A. Freeman (eds.), *The Computerization of Behavioral Healthcare: How to Enhance Clinical Practice, Management, and Communications.* San Francisco: Jossey-Bass, 1996.

Slack, W. V., Van Cura, L. J., and Greist, J. H. "Computers and Doctors: Use and Consequences." *Computers and Biomedical Research,* 1970, *3,* 521–527.

Zieman, Y. L., and Bleich, H. L. "Conceptual Mapping of User's Queries to Medical Subject Headings." *Proceedings of the American Medical Informatics Association,* 1997, 519–522.

Chapter Ten (Confidentiality)

Aronson, M. D. "Catch-22 in the Era of Peer Review Organizations." *M.D. Computing,* 1992, *9*(5), 284–285.

Barber, B. "Current Issues in Data Protection." *Medical Informatics (London),* 1989, *14,* 207–209.

Barrows, R. C., Jr., and Clayton, P. D. "Privacy, Confidentiality, and Electronic Medical Records." *Journal of the American Medical Informatics Association,* 1996, *3*(2), 139–149.

Bleich, H. L. "Sidney R. Garfield and the Crisis in Health Care." *M.D. Computing,* 1994, *11*(1), 5–6.

Bleich, H. L., Beckley, R. F., Horowitz, G., Jackson, J., Moody, E., Franklin, C., Goodman, S. R., McKay, M. W., Pope, R. A., Walden, T., Bloom, S. A., and Slack, W. V. "Clinical Computing in a Teaching Hospital." *New England Journal of Medicine,* 1985, *312*(12), 756–764.

Bleich, H. L., Safran, C., and Slack, W. V. "Departmental and Laboratory Computing in Two Hospitals." *M.D. Computing,* 1989, *6*(3), 149–155.

Brannigan, V. M. "Patient Privacy: A Consumer Protection Approach." *Journal of Medical Systems,* 1984, *8,* 501–505.

Day, N. M. "Medical Information Bureau Report." *Transactions of the American Academy of Insurance Medicine Annual Meeting,* 1993, *76,* 18–20.

Entmacher, P. S. "Medical Information Bureau." *Journal of the American Medical Association,* 1975, *233*(13), 1370–1372.

Garfield, S. R. "The Delivery of Medical Care." *Scientific American,* 1970, *222,* 15–23.

Gritzalis, D., Katsikas, S., Keklikoglou, J., and Tomaras, A. "Data Security in Medical Information Systems: Technical Aspects of a Proposed Legislation." *Medical Informatics (London),* 1991, *16,* 371–383.

Hiatt, H. H. *America's Health Care in the Balance: Choice or Chance.* New York: HarperCollins, 1987.

Kassirer, J. P. "Managed Care and the Morality of the Marketplace." *New England Journal of Medicine,* 1995, *333,* 50–52.

Rind, D. M., Kohane, I. S., Szolovits, P., Safran, C., Chueh, H. C., and Barnett, G. O. "Maintaining the Confidentiality of Medical Records Shared Over the Internet and the World Wide Web." *Annals of Internal Medicine,* 1997, *127,* 138–141.

Robinson, E. N., Jr. "The Computerized Patient Record: Privacy and Security." *M.D. Computing,* 1994, *11*(2), 69–73.

Rosenberg, C. E. *The Care of Strangers: The Rise of America's Hospital System.* New York: Basic Books, 1987.

Rothfeder, J. *Privacy for Sale: How Computerization Has Made Everyone's Private Life an Open Secret.* New York: Simon & Schuster, 1992.

Safran, C., Porter, D., Lightfoot, J., Rury, C. D., Underhill, L. H., Bleich, H. L., and Slack, W. V. "ClinQuery: A System for On-line Searching of Data in a Teaching Hospital." *Annals of Internal Medicine,* 1989, *9,* 751–756.

Safran, C., Rind, D., Citroen, M., Bakker, A. R., Slack, W. V., and Bleich, H. L.

"Protection of Confidentiality in the Computer-Based Patient Record." *M.D. Computing,* 1995, *12*(3), 187–192.

Safran, C., Rury, C., Rind, D. M., and Taylor, W. C. "A Computer-Based Ambulatory Medical Record for a Teaching Hospital." *M.D. Computing,* 1991, *8*(5), 291–299.

Safran, C., Slack, W. V., and Bleich, H. L. "Role of Computing in Patient Care in Two Hospitals." *M.D. Computing,* 1989, *6*(3), 141–148.

Shea, S. "Security Versus Access: Trade-Offs Are Only Part of the Story." *Journal of the American Medical Informatics Association,* 1994, *1,* 314–315.

Slack, W. V. "Patient Power." In J. A. Jacquez (ed.), *Computer Diagnosis and Diagnostic Methods: The Proceedings of the Second Conference on the Diagnostic Process Held at the University of Michigan.* Springfield, Ill.: Thomas, 1972.

Slack, W. V. "The Issue of Privacy." *M.D. Computing,* 1997, *14,* 8–11.

Slack, W. V. "Private Information in the Hands of Strangers." *M.D. Computing,* 1997, *14,* 83–86.

Slee, V., Slee, D., and Schmidt, H. J. *The Endangered Medical Record: Ensuring Its Integrity in the Age of Informatics.* Saint Paul, Minn.: Tringa Press, 2000.

Van der Leer, O. F. "The Use of Personal Data for Medical Research: How to Deal with New European Privacy Standards." *International Journal of Biomedical Computing,* 1994, *35*(Suppl.), 87–95.

Wald, J. S., Rind D., and Safran, C. "Protecting Confidentiality in an Electronic Medical Record: Feedback to the Author When Someone Reads a Clinical Note." *American Medical Informatics Association Spring Proceedings,* 1994.

Weed, L. L. "Medical Records That Guide and Teach." *New England Journal of Medicine,* 1968, *278,* 593–600, 652–657.

Weingarten, J. "Can Confidential Information Be Kept Private in High-Tech Medicine?" *M.D. Computing,* 1992, *9*(2), 79–82.

Chapter Eleven (Barriers to Cybermedicine)

Bleich, H. L. "The Computer as a Consultant." *New England Journal of Medicine,* 1971, *284,* 141–147.

Bleich, H. L. "Charles Babbage and His Steam-Driven Computer." *M.D. Computing,* 1992, 9(2), 6–10.

Bleich, H. L. "Why Good Hospitals Get Bad Computing." In B. Cesnik, A. T. McCray, and J. R. Scherrer (eds.), *MEDINFO '98.* Amsterdam: IOS Press, 1998.

Brennan, P. F., Ripich, S., and Moore, S. M. "The Use of Home-Based Computers to Support Persons Living with AIDS/ARC." *Journal of Community Health Nursing,* 1991, *8*(1), 3–14.

Flatley-Brennan, P. "Computer Network Home Care Demonstration: A Randomized Trial in Persons Living with AIDS." *Computers in Biology and Medicine,* 1998, *28,* 489–508.

Gustafson, D. H., Bosworth, K., Hawkins, R. P., Boberg, E. W., and Bricker, E. "CHESS: A Computer-Based System for Providing Information, Referrals, Decision Support and Social Support to People Facing Medical and Other Health-Related Crises." In M. E. Frisse (ed.), *Proceedings of the Sixteenth Annual Symposium on Computer Applications in Medical Care.* Baltimore, Md.: American Medical Informatics Association, 1992.

Gustafson, D. H., Hawkins, R. P., Boberg, E. W., Bricker, E., Pingree, S., and Chan, C. L. "The Use and Impact of a Computer-Based Support System for People Living with AIDS and HIV Infection." In J. G. Ozbolt (ed.), *Proceedings of the Eighteenth Annual Symposium on Computer Applications in Medical Care.* Washington, D.C.: American Medical Informatics Association, 1994.

Gustafson, D. H., Hawkins, R., Boberg, E., Pingree, S., Serlin, R. E., Graziano, F., and Chan, C. L. "Impact of a Patient-Centered, Computer-Based Health Information/Support System." *American Journal of Preventive Medicine,* 1999, *16,* 1–9.

McTavish, F. M., Gustafson, D. H., Owens, B. H., Hawkins, R. P., Pingree, S., Wise, M., Taylor, J. O., and Apantaku, F. M. "CHESS (Comprehensive Health Enhancement Support System), an Interactive Computer System for Women with Breast Cancer Piloted with an Underserved Population." *Journal of Ambulatory Care Management,* 1995, *18*(3), 35–41.

Nader, R. *Unsafe at Any Speed: The Designed-in Dangers of the American Automobile.* New York: Grossman, 1965.

Parkinson, C. N. *Parkinson's Law.* New York: Ballantine, 1987.

Shaw, B. R., McTavish, F., Hawkins, R., Gustafson, D. H., and Pingree, S. "Experiences of Women with Breast Cancer: Exchanging Social Support Over the CHESS Computer Network." *Journal of Health Community,* 2000, *5,* 135–159.

Skinner, B. F. *The Behavior of Organisms: An Experimental Analysis.* Englewood Cliffs, N.J.: Appleton-Century-Crofts, 1938.

Slack, W. V. "Use of Computers." In *MEDINFO '80, Proceedings of the Third World Conference on Medical Informatics.* Amsterdam: 1980.

Slack, W. V. "The Soul of a New System: a Modern Parable." *Massachusetts Medicine,* 1987, *2,* 24–28.

Slack, W. V. "A Brief Treatise on the Academic Committee." *M.D. Computing,* 1990, *7*(5), 282–284.

Slack, W. V. "Type 1 and Type 2 Administrators." *M.D. Computing,* 1990, *7*(2), 69–70.

Slack, W. V. "The Forces of Bureaucracy." *M.D. Computing,* 1992, *9*(3), 133–135.

Slack, W. V. "When the Machine Stops." *M.D. Computing,* 1992, *9*(1), 6–10.

Slack, W. V., and Bleich, H. L. "The CCC System in Two Teaching Hospitals: A Progress Report." *International Journal of Medical Informatics,* 1999, *54,* 183–196.

Slack, W. V., Boro, E. S., and Bleich, H. L. "Barriers to Clinical Computing: What Physicians Can Do." *M.D. Computing,* 1992, *9*(5), 278–280.

Slack, W. V., Van Cura, L. J., and Greist, J. H. "Computers and Doctors: Use and Consequences." *Computers and Biomedical Research,* 1970, *3,* 521–527.

Von Neumann, J. *The Computer and the Brain.* New Haven, Conn.: Yale University Press, 1958.

Watson, J. B. *Behaviorism.* New York: Norton, 1924.

Woolhandler, S., Himmelstein, D. U., and Lewontin, J. P. "Administrative Costs in U.S. Hospitals." *New England Journal of Medicine,* 1993, *329,* 400–403.

Chapter Twelve (The Importance of Being Ernst)

Bleich, H. L. "Why Good Hospitals Get Bad Computing." In B. Cesnik, A. T. McCray, and J. R. Scherrer (eds.), *MEDINFO '98.* Amsterdam: IOS Press, 1998.

Parkinson, C. N. *Parkinson's Law.* New York: Ballantine, 1987.

Slack, W. V. "The Soul of a New System: A Modern Parable." *Massachusetts Medicine,* 1987, *2,* 24–28.

Slack, W. V. "A Brief Treatise on the Academic Committee." *M.D. Computing,* 1990, *7*(5), 282–284.

Slack, W. V. "Type 1 and Type 2 Administrators." *M.D. Computing,* 1990, *7*(2), 69–70.

Slack, W. V. "The Forces of Bureaucracy." *M.D. Computing,* 1992, *9*(3), 133–135.

Chapter Thirteen (New Horizons)

Blignault, I. "Multipoint Videoconferencing in Health: A Review of Three Years' Experience in Queensland, Australia." *Telemedicine Journal,* 2000, *6,* 269–274.

Eng, T. R., Maxfield, A., Paatrick, K., Deering, M. J., Ratzan, S. C., and Gustafson, D. H. "Access to Health Information and Support: A Public Highway or a Private Road?" *Journal of the American Medical Association,* 1998, *280,* 1371–1375.

Feinstein, A. R. "Twentieth Century Paradigms That Threaten Both Scientific and Humane Medicine in the Twenty-First Century." *Journal of Clinical Epidemiology,* 1996, *49,* 615–617.

Goldberg, M. A. "Teleradiology and Telemedicine." *Radiology Clinics of North America,* 1996, *34*(3), 647–665.

Gray, J. E., Safran, C., Davis, R. B., Pompilio-Weitzner, G., Stewart, J. E., Zaccagnini, L., and Pursley, D. "Baby CareLink: Using the Internet and Telemedicine to Improve Care for High-Risk Infants." *Pediatrics,* 2000, *106,* 1318–1324.

Hiatt, H. H. *America's Health Care in the Balance: Choice or Chance.* New York: HarperCollins, 1987.

Kane, B., and Sands, D. Z. "Guidelines for the Clinical Use of Electronic Mail with Patients." *Journal of the American Medical Informatics Association,* 1998, *5,* 104–111.

Lenert, L. A. "Use of Meta-Analytic Results to Facilitate Shared Decision Making." *Journal of the American Medical Informatics Association,* 1999, *6*(5), 412–419.

Mair, F. S., Haycox, A., May, C., and Williams, T. "A Review of Telemedicine Cost-Effectiveness Studies." *Journal of Telemedicine Telecare,* 2000, *6*(Supplement 1), S38-S40.

Mulley, A. G. "Supporting the Patient's Role in Decision Making." *Journal of Occupational Medicine,* 1990, *32*(12), 1227–1228.

Miller, R. A., Schaffner, K. F., and Meisel, A. "Ethical and Legal Issues Related to the Use of Computer Programs in Clinical Medicine." *Annals of Internal Medicine,* 1985, *102,* 529–537.

Slack, W. V., Boro, E. S., and Bleich, H. L. "Barriers to Clinical Computing: What Physicians Can Do." *M.D. Computing,* 1992, *9*(5), 278–280.

Epilogue

de Tocqueville, A. *Democracy in America.* (G. Lawrence, trans.). Garden City, N.Y.: Doubleday, 1969. (Originally published 1835, 1840.)

Forster, E. M. "The Machine Stops." In *The Eternal Moment and Other Stories.* Orlando: Harcourt Brace, 1928.

Slack, W. V. "When the Machine Stops." *M.D. Computing,* 1992, *9*(1), 6–10.

Slack, W. V. "When the Home Is Also the Clinic." *M.D. Computing,* 1996, *13*(6), 465–468.

—*∿*— **About the Author**

Dr. Slack received his bachelor's degree from Princeton University, his medical degree from Columbia University's College of Physicians and Surgeons, and his residency training in neurology at the University of Wisconsin. Over the past thirty-five years he has focused his research on the use of computers to improve communication in medicine and to empower both doctors and patients for better health care. His early work in computer-based medical interviewing at the University of Wisconsin led to the first study of patient-computer dialogue. Over the years, he has established new computer-based approaches to the medical interview and has developed and studied programs that provide direct assistance to the patient in the management of common, important medical and psychological problems. He was an early advocate of the patients' right to participate as partners with their clinicians in decisions about diagnosis and treatment.

During the past twenty years, Dr. Slack and his colleagues at the Center for Clinical Computing (CCC) and the Harvard Medical School have developed, implemented, and studied an integrated, hospital-wide cybermedicine system (the CCC system), which is used in patient care at Boston's Beth Israel Deaconess Medical Center and Brigham and Women's Hospital. A distinguishing feature of the CCC system is the unparalleled intensity and extensiveness of its use by clinicians in the care of their patients.

Pursuing his interest in the field of mental testing, Dr. Slack has examined the use and misuse of the Scholastic Aptitude Test, and the results of his studies, done in collaboration with Dr. Douglas Porter, have been influential in reformative efforts, such as the "truth in testing" legislation in New York State.

Dr. Slack is professor of medicine and psychiatry at Harvard Medical School and, with Dr. Howard L. Bleich, copresident of the Center for Clinical Computing and codirector of the Division of Clinical Computing, Department of Medicine, Beth Israel Deaconess Medical Center.

~~~ Index

DATE DUE